HOW MANY DOCTORS DO WE NEED?

How Many Doctors Do We Need?

A Policy Agenda for the United States in the 1990s

Based on the Tenth Private Sector Conference, 1985

Edited by Duncan Yaggy and Patricia Hodgson

Foreword by William G. Anlyan

Duke Press Policy Studies

Duke University Press   Durham, 1986

© 1986 Duke University Press
All rights reserved
Printed in the United States of America
on acid-free paper ∞
Library of Congress Cataloging in Publication Data
appear at the end of this book.

Contents

Foreword / WILLIAM G. ANLYAN   ix
Participants   x

1

Overview of Public and Private Policies
Affecting Physician Supply in the U.S. / WILLIAM G. ANLYAN   1
Legislative Perspective / PAUL G. ROGERS   9
Historical Perspective / ROSEMARY A. STEVENS   11
GMENAC Revisited / ALVIN R. TARLOV   13
The Physician Surplus: Another View / WILLIAM B. SCHWARTZ   19
Market Forces and Geographic Distribution of Physicians /
JOSEPH P. NEWHOUSE   23
Correcting "Surpluses" and "Shortages" in Medical Specialties
    I.   The Surgeons / C. ROLLINS HANLON   28
    II.   The Physicians / ROBERT H. MOSER   30
Life-style Choices and Evolving Practice Patterns /
BRITAIN NICHOLSON   34
Market Influences of FMGS / SAMUEL P. ASPER   37
Methodological Problems in Assessing Physician Demand, Need,
and Supply: Policy Implications / UWE E. REINHARDT   41
Discussion   46

2

The University's Role in Establishing Priorities for Medical
Education—A Societal Perspective / WILLIAM H. DANFORTH   55

Managing Quality and Quantity in Residency Training Programs /
JOHN S. GRAETTINGER   60

The Impact of State Licensing Boards on the Distribution and
Quality of Physicians / BRYANT L. GALUSHA   64

The Experience in Great Britain / JOHN LISTER   70

Discussion   80

3
Public and Private Options for Assessing and Managing Physician
Manpower Supply / ROBERT G. PETERSDORF   97

Comments
   I.   From the AAMC/ JOHN A. D. COOPER   106
   II. From the AMA / JAMES H. SAMMONS   109
   III. From a Private Medical School / DANIEL C. TOSTESON   112
   IV. From a Public Medical School / M. ROY SCHWARZ   115
   V. Third-party Payment: Industry / WILLIS GOLDBECK   118
   VI. Law / CLARK C. HAVIGHURST   124
   VII. State Government / EUGENE S. MAYER   127

Discussion   134

4
Summary
   I.   Alain C. Enthoven   147
   II. Arnold S. Relman   152
   III. J. Alexander McMahon   155

Index   157

Figures and Tables

Figures

1. Medicine Evolves into a Science, 1846–1909   2
2. Post-Flexner to World War II, 1910–44   3
3. Post–World War II Era: Sputnik and Social Justice, 1945–65   4
4. Medicare/Medicaid and the Great Society to an Age of Limited Resources, 1965–85   5
5. Ratio M.D.s/Population   7
6. Physician Diffusion as Supply Grows: Towns of 5,000, 10,000 and 30,000 Population   23
7. A Simple Forecasting Equation for Physician Manpower   42
8. An Economic Definition of a Physician Surplus   44
9. Ratio of Physicians to Applicants and the Number of Unmatched Applicants   61
10. Positions Available, by Category, Filled by U.S. Senior Students   62
11. Doctor/Population Quotient in Great Britain   72
12. Career Structure   73
13. Hospital Staff: England and Wales   74
14. Numbers of Doctors in Each Grade by Place of Birth: England and Wales   75
15. Applications and Acceptances for Medical Schools, 1983   78
16. Growth in Numbers of Junior Doctors and Consultants: Great Britain, 1970–79   79
17. Specialty Distribution   102
18. Percentage of Residents by Specialty, 1983   103
19. Physician/10,000 Population Ratio for Nonmetropolitan Counties in North Carolina and the United States, 1979–80   129
20. Change in Physician/Population Ratio by County, 1963–83   130

21. Counties Served by the North Carolina Area Health
     Education Centers Program   131

Tables

1. Average Number of Office Visits per Year by Gender of
    Physician: Internal Medicine, United States, 1981   43
2. Differentials in Workload of Men and Women Physicians
    in Private Practice: France, 1981   43

Foreword

For the Tenth Private Sector Conference we chose a topic that troubles physicians, educators, and policymakers: the growing supply of physicians in the United States. We focused on two questions: Is there a surplus of physicians now, or in prospect? If there is, what should be done about it, if anything?

The conferees expressed a variety of strong opinions on these questions. All the participants agreed that the growing supply of physicians will have a significant impact on American health care, and on physicians themselves, but they could not agree what the impact will be and whether it will be beneficial or detrimental. There was general agreement that the rapidly increasing influx of new physicians from foreign medical schools posed a serious threat, but a proposal to curtail the flow produced sharp controversy.

We agreed on little, but our discussions gave all of us a better understanding of the issues and their significance. And that, after all, is the true purpose of the Private Sector Conference.

On behalf of the conferees, I would like to thank the Duke University Medical Center, the Duke Endowment, and the American Medical Association for the support that made the conference possible.

W. G. Anlyan, M.D.
Chancellor for Health Affairs
Duke University

Participants

JOHN E. AFFELDT, M.D., President, Joint Commission on Accreditation of Hospitals

WILLIAM G. ANLYAN, M.D., Chancellor for Health Affairs, Duke University

SAMUEL P. ASPER, M.D., President, Education Commission for Foreign Medical Graduates

JOSEPH F. BOYLE, M.D., President, American Medical Association

JOHN W. COLLOTON, Director and Assistant to the President for Statewide Health Services, University of Iowa Hospitals and Clinics

JOHN A. D. COOPER, M.D., President, Association of American Medical Colleges

WILLIAM H. DANFORTH, M.D. Chancellor, Washington University

C. DOUGLAS EAVENSON, Assistant Director, Employee Benefits and Services, General Motors Corporation

RICHARD H. EGDAHL, M.D., Academic Vice President and Director of the Medical Center, Boston University

PAUL M. ELLWOOD, JR., M.D., President, Interstudy

ALAIN C. ENTHOVEN, Ph.D., Mariner S. Eccles Professor of Public and Private Management, Stanford University

HARVEY V. FINEBERG, M.D., Dean, Harvard School of Public Health

ASHLEY H. GALE, JR., Director, Hospital and Child Care Division, The Duke Endowment

BRYANT L. GALUSHA, M.D., Executive Vice President, Federation of State Medical Boards

ELI GINZBERG, Ph.D., Director, Conservation of Human Resources, Columbia University

WILLIS GOLDBECK, President, Washington Business Group on Health

JOHN S. GRAETTINGER, M.D., Associate Dean, Graduate Medical Education, St. Luke's Medical Center

C. ROLLINS HANLON, M.D., Director, American College of Surgeons

CLARK C. HAVIGHURST, J.D., School of Law, Duke University

JOHN LISTER, M.D., Postgraduate Dean, British Postgraduate Medical Foundation, University of London

BILLY G. MCCALL, Deputy Executive Director and Secretary, The Duke Endowment

J. ALEXANDER MCMAHON, President, American Hospital Association

MARGARET MAHONEY, President, The Commonwealth Fund

EUGENE S. MAYER, M.D., Associate Dean, AHEC Program Director, University of North Carolina

ROBERT H. MOSER, M.D., Executive Vice President, American College of Physicians

TOM E. NESBITT, M.D., Urology Associates, Nashville, Tennessee

JOSEPH P. NEWHOUSE, Ph.D., Chief, Economic Department, Rand Corporation

BRITAIN NICHOLSON, M.D., Boston, Massachusetts

DAVID J. OTTENSMEYER, M.D., President, Lovelace Medical Foundation

ROBERT G. PETERSDORF, M.D., Vice Chancellor and Dean, School of Medicine, University of California

UWE E. REINHARDT, Ph.D., James Madison Professor of Political Economy, Woodrow Wilson School of Public & International Affairs, Princeton University

ARNOLD S. RELMAN, M.D., Editor, *New England Journal of Medicine*

B. L. RHODES, Executive Vice President, Kaiser Foundation Health Plan, Inc.

PAUL G. ROGERS, Attorney at Law, Hogan & Hartson Law Firm

JAMES H. SAMMONS, M.D., Executive Vice President, American Medical Association

DAVID SATCHER, M.D., Ph.D., President, Meharry Medical College

WILLIAM B. SCHWARTZ, M.D., Vannevar Bush University Professor and Professor of Medicine, Tufts University

M. Roy Schwarz, M.D., Vice President, Medical Education and Science Policy, American Medical Association

Jack K. Shelton, Manager, Employee Insurance Department, Ford Motor Company

Rosemary A. Stevens, Ph.D., Professor, Department of History and Sociology of Science, University of Pennsylvania

Alvin R. Tarlov, M.D., President, Henry J. Kaiser Family Foundation

Daniel C. Tosteson, M.D., Dean, Harvard Medical School

Edwin C. Whitehead, Chairman, Whitehead Associates

Richard S. Wilbur, M.D., Executive Vice President, Council of Medical Specialty Societies

Jere Witherspoon, Associate Director, Hospital and Child Care Division, The Duke Endowment

Rita Wroblewski, Ph.D., Director of Medical Affairs, Pfizer, Inc.

John Iglehart, Rapporteur

I

Overview of Public and Private Policies Affecting Physician Supply in the United States

WILLIAM G. ANLYAN, M.D.

First and foremost, we must define what physicians are all about. I choose to say that the basic mission of physicians is to improve the health care of the people they serve. Physicians' services are neither a commodity nor a luxury; rather they provide basic needs for the prevention and cure of disease and the alleviation of suffering.

In colonial times, most of the physicians in this country were trained in Great Britain, particularly Edinburgh and London. The first controls in medicine came in with the licensing boards in New York in 1760, which were followed by the founding of the first College of Medicine in Philadelphia in 1765, which became the University of Pennsylvania; the founding of Harvard Medical School in 1783; and then Kings College, which became Columbia, in 1792.

Interwoven from this point on in this overview of medicine in the United States are the major scientific discoveries and events that have affected the numbers of doctors and the quality of health care. In 1809 the first quasi-elective laparotomy was done in Kentucky by Ephraim McDowell. A woman rode on horseback for sixty miles to have a 22.5 pound tumor removed from her abdomen on a kitchen table without anesthesia.

In 1810 Yale Medical School was founded and then came the Jacksonian era of deregulation in the 1830s, leading from four medical schools to thirty by 1840 and to seventy-seven by 1876. During this era of deregulation came the discovery of anesthesia, initially by Crawford Long in 1843, and then the ether dome demonstration at Massachusetts General Hospital (MGH) in 1846. Figure 1 shows medical history from this point until 1909. The American Medical Association (AMA) was founded in 1847 to

Figure 1. Medicine Evolves into a Science, 1846–1909.

1846	Anesthesia: Long vs. Morton
1847	AMA founded
1864	Specialty societies started; American Ophthalmological Society
1876	AAMC founded
1871–77	Harvard medical reform
	Pasteur, Lister, Koch
1893	Johns Hopkins
1895	Discovery of x-ray: Dr. Roentgen
1901	Landsteiner
1905	160 medical schools, 5,600 graduates
1907	AMA: CME

bring some professional order to medicine. Then the specialty societies evolved, starting with the ophthalmologists in 1864 and the Association of American Medical Colleges (AAMC) in 1876. At about the same time we had the work of Pasteur, Lister, and Koch leading to antisepsis and bacteriology.

Harvard Medical School underwent its reform in the 1870s under President Eliott, over the near-dead body of the Chief of Surgery, Henry Bigelow, at the MGH. Eliott wanted all students to know how to read and write, and Bigelow thought that that would restrict their admissions pool.

In 1893 came another very definite milestone, the founding of Johns Hopkins, the model on which many other schools of medicine have been based. In 1895 the discovery of x-ray occurred, and in 1901 Landsteiner performed the first blood transfusion. In 1905 there were 160 medical schools and 5,600 graduates. In 1907 the AMA formed the Council on Medical Education to focus on the problems of medical education within that organization. During the early 1900s medicine evolved into a science as opposed to the previous era of *purgare et sangare,* which Molière described as all that physicians could do for their patients: bleed and purge.

With the aid of the Carnegie Corporation, Abraham Flexner in 1910 (figure 2) did his study of the quality of medical education, resulting in the closing of many of the second- and third-rate medical colleges of the time.

In 1912 the College of Surgeons and the College of Physicians were formed and in 1915 came the beginning of the specialty boards for examination. By 1920 the number of medical schools had shrunk from 160 to 60, and the movement in the country was toward increasing specialization. There were fewer and fewer physicians in rural areas and the poor were not sufficiently cared for. Such foundations as the Rockefeller and subsequently the Duke Endowment became concerned and encouraged the formation of new medical schools.

In 1924 insulin was discovered, prolonging the lives of subsequent diabetics. But in 1930 the AMA and the AAMC began to suggest that we were creating too many medical schools, and in 1934 the president of the AMA suggested closing half of the schools. Shortly thereafter, in the AAMC setting, Arthur Dean Bevan suggested that we cut down on admissions by 5 percent and increase the requirements for licensure. This occurred at the same time that third-party insurance was creeping in and the sulfa drugs were coming into use.

In 1937 Weiskotten, heading a statesmanlike commission, suggested leaving the numbers of medical students alone but improving their quality. In 1941 the United States entered World War II and needed more doctors, so classes were accelerated with a net gain of perhaps one or one and one-half classes. During the war, penicillin was discovered and some control of microbacterial infections began.

Figure 2. Post-Flexner to World War II, 1910–44.

1910	Carnegie: Flexner
1912	Colleges
1915	Specialty boards
1920	60 schools
1920–24	Foundations encourage new schools
	Increasing specialization
	Decreasing numbers of rural M.D.s
	Decline in the care of the poor
1924	Insulin
1930	AMA and AAMC: ? too many
1934	AMA (Bierring): close half of the schools
1934–37	Third-party insurance
	Sulfa drugs
1936	AAMC (Bevan): admissions decline 5%, licensing increases
1937	Weiskotten: quality improves
1941	World War II: increased need for M.D.s, accelerated classes
1944	Penicillin

In 1945 (figure 3) the NIH evolved from the adolescent unit that existed at that time, and in 1948 the Hill-Burton Act was enacted, creating rural hospitals. New VA hospitals were created in juxtaposition to universities. And the AAMC declared that we needed to double medical school enrollment.

If somebody had asked me in 1948 what kind of hospital I thought we should build for the next decade, I would have said we need more tuberculosis hospitals and more polio hospitals and convalescent centers. Yet we see from the vantage point of some years later that tuberculosis was coming under control and research in the next few years would lead to the polio vaccine. By 1949–50 the Truman Commission tended to agree with the AAMC about the need for more doctors but the AMA raised the question of whether the data were good enough to support those suggestions. The AMA preferred to leave it to the universities to decide about class size; they were accused of trying to protect the physician's income at that time and nothing much happened. In the four-year period between 1952–56, the number of foreign medical graduates (FMGs) multiplied fourfold.

Figure 3. Post-World War II Era: Sputnik and Social Justice, 1945–65.

1945	NIH
1948	Hill-Burton Act
	VA-university relationships
	AAMC: need to double enrollment
1952	Magnuson and Truman: same
	AMA: ? data and leave to university
	? to protect M.D. income
	FMGs quadruple in four years
	Tuberculosis declines
1956	Little Rock
	Polio
1957	Sputnik
	Heart disease on the rise
1959	Civil Rights movement; increased attempts to solve social problems through government
	AMA and AAMC agree on need to increase numbers of schools and M.D.s
	Transplantation
1963	First HPEA Act: construction, loans B.I.G.
	HPEA revisions: need 50% more M.D.s within a decade
1965	Coggeshall and Millis (AAMC)

Figure 4. Medicare/Medicaid and the Great Society to an Age of Limited
Resources, 1965–85.

1965	Medicare/Medicaid
1969	P.A.P.: increases 10%
1970	Carnegie Commission: 50% increase, and increased federal aid
1971	Health Manpower Act: capitation bonus increases, new schools, convert 2-year schools to 4-year schools
1972	National HS Corps: geographic maldistribution
1973	Weinberger
1975	70,000 more FMGS: one-third I and R; one-fifth U.S. M.D.s HPEA + U.S. FMGS (decreased one year later) SOSSUS
1976	AHECS GMENAC (1976–80)
1978	IOM: no increase
1981	Capitation kaput

Then came the Little Rock incident in 1956, which completely blurred what happened in Hungary, and in 1957 the Sputnik, followed by a great movement to increase the civil rights of our citizens and solve social problems through governmental action. Shortly thereafter, both the AMA and the AAMC agreed upon the need to increase the number of medical schools and the enrollment of physicians. Together they persuaded the federal government to write the first Health Professions Educational Act for the construction of new schools and the expansion of existing schools, for loans, and for basic improvement grants. A year later this was in federal legislation.

In 1965 the Coggeshall report supported the expansion of medical education and the Millis Commission of the AMA threw its support to the creation of family practice as a specialty. This period brought the evolution of the treatment of heart disease and the beginnings of transplantation of kidneys and other organs in the laboratory.

We come to the era of Medicare and Medicaid and the Great Society (figure 4) and its evolution into the age of limited resources. In 1965 the legislation for Medicare/Medicaid was passed. In 1969 the Nixon Administration asked for a physician augmentation program, increasing the enrollment of physicians by 10 percent within nine months. In 1970 the Carnegie Commission suggested a 50 percent increase in the enrollment and an increase in federal aid. In 1971 there was another Health Manpower Act with a capitation bonus and clauses to increase medical school size and to convert two-year medical schools to four-year schools. Because of the geographic maldistribution of our population, the National Health Service Corps was also established.

In 1973 Caspar Weinberger, then Secretary of the Department of Health, Education, and Welfare, suggested there were too many future physicians in the pipeline. By 1975 there were over 70,000 foreign medical graduates (FMGS) in the system; one-third of the interns and residents were foreign medical graduates and one-fifth of practicing U.S. physicians came from abroad. Shortly thereafter, the renewal of the Health Professions Educational Assistance Act suggested that all schools had to absorb a certain number of American FMGS from Guadalajara and the Caribbean Basin, but there was such a hullabaloo that the provision was dropped a year later.

In 1975 a study of the surgical services of the United States began looking at the different types of surgeons and whether there was an excess or a shortage. A year later area health education centers, one of the suggestions of the Carnegie Commission, were developed. Between 1976 and 1980 the GMENAC Commission came out with its suggestion that we did indeed have a major surplus of doctors coming down the pipeline. In 1978 the Institute of Medicine suggested maintaining the status quo. By 1981 the capitation program had ended; no longer did we get federal support for our medical schools in that form.

The physician/population ratio is another way to consider the question of physician excess or shortage. Prior to 1980 the physician/population ratio was highest in 1850 (figure 5), when there was one physician for every 571 people. In 1980 there was one for every 465 people. If you eliminate part-time practicing physicians, there was one for every 520 people.

Now let us look at the major forces facing a change of any kind: the aging population will have to be considered in our recommendations, as will the declining birthrate, which is already reflected in the number of applicants to medical schools; the change in the economy from the Great Society of 1965, where more was better and the approach was open-ended, to selection and substituted choices of what the country can do; the unknowns in the scientific breakthroughs that will prevent the polios and cure the tuberculoses; the tremendous ability of our colleagues to produce bigger and better and more complex halfway technologies in trans-

Figure 5. Ratio M.D.s/Population.

	M.D.s	Population	Ratio
1850	40,755	23,261,000	1/571
1860	55,055	31,513,000	1/572
1870	64,414	39,905,000	1/619
1880	85,671	50,262,000	1/587
1890	100,180	63,056,000	1/629
1900	119,749	76,094,000	1/635
1910	135,000	92,407,000	1/684
1920	144,797	106,461,000	1/735
1930	153,803	123,188,000	1/800
1940	175,163	132,122,000	1/754
1950	203,400	151,684,000	1/745
1960	274,833	180,671,000	1/657
1970	348,328	204,879,000	1/588
1980	487,000	226,346,000	1/465

Sources: Historical Statistics of the United States Colonial Times to 1790;
Statistical Abstract of the United States, 1984.

plantation and heart disease and unknown progress in brain research and in the newer sciences just around the corner; and the increasing number of procedures available to nonsurgeons in the system at the present time.

Other major forces are: the increasing number of women in medicine, which has brought a very fine change in sensitivity in medicine; the changing life-styles of our future physicians and younger physicians; the political force of USFMGS — we know how strong they are from what happened in the late seventies; the increasing political base of foreign medical graduates; the AMA, the AAMC, the Colleges, and the Boards; the AHA looming as a very major force in graduate medical education, which, to me, is the center of the continuum of continuing medical education today; the states, the federal government, and the business world, which some have dubbed the fourth party at the present time — a very major force; and the third-party insurers who are no longer a pass-through but who are getting into the act of policy decisions.

My tentative conclusion in looking at the past is that the United States is a heterogeneous country with an open system of health care. We have a powerful private sector using influence, persuasion, and market economics and not solely government decree. Forty percent of our health care is government controlled; added to that is the va system. Yet the responsiveness of medical care and health care is less dominated by a central government and its politics than is true in other developed nations.

The U.S. health care system is a multisystem. Breakthroughs in biomedical research impact significantly at an accelerating rate. The only major gap in this multisystem is the health care of the uninsured poor. There have been sharp swings of the pendulum regarding whether we have too many doctors or too few. It is obvious that when the aamc and the ama row together—particularly if they pull in the foundations and government—the system tends to change.

So the questions we face among others are: acknowledging the historic pendulum swings of opinion and the unforeseen breakthroughs of biomedical research, do we have a looming major physician surplus? Do we have a continuing uneven specialty and geographic distribution? If there are imbalances, should the corrections be addressed by universities, other private sector forces, the state or the federal government, or a combination thereof?

Our ultimate objective in seeking a fair, unbiased trend in manpower development must be to provide appropriate, high-quality medical care for all Americans.

Legislative Perspective
PAUL G. ROGERS

It is true that the Congress perceived a need for an increase in health manpower in the early 1970s. When a national need exists, the Congress usually reacts, as it did in this situation, with hearings and investigations, trying to bring before itself and the public experts to educate the nation on the problem. Many studies, the Carnegie as well as others, developed evidence that there was a shortage of some 40,000 to 50,000 doctors, and shortages of dentists and nurses as well. The AAMC spearheaded the effort to alleviate this shortage, and I recall no significant groups that opposed the health manpower legislation. It was the general consensus of the scientific and medical groups that something needed to be done.

While Congress often reacts to testimony from experts, that does not necessarily get the legislation passed. What really gets legislation passed is the fact that those congressmen and senators hear from their constituents at home about what is happening in their states and districts; in this case, example after example of shortages came forth from those districts and from the states. Some communities were advertising to get a doctor to come to their community. Many offered to build an office for them, build a clinic or even a hospital, and the Congress heard this. They heard that many people couldn't get their needs met in their areas. In some rather affluent areas doctors were taking no new patients. Without question, the need for more physicians existed. This was not just a perceived need but an actual need, and the Congress was convinced about it.

At the time we were considering health manpower, medical schools often had to use the fiction of getting research grants for their staff, although the research dollars often were used to support the educational activities of the medical schools. There was no other source of those dollars for education. It was the capitation program that finally supported education for education's sake so that the professor didn't have to go to the research application to maintain himself and his activity.

We were also beginning to set up distress grants at that time, and some sixty medical colleges made application for distress grants. Without question the need was well established, the Congress acted, and the medical universities responded in a magnificent way.

Today things are changing so rapidly that before we come to a quick conclusion that we are going to have too many doctors we should look at the situation very carefully. If, for example, the Veterans Administration undergoes the change that has been proposed in taking care of veterans, a vast number of veterans will come back to the private sector for medical care. The Congress is now considering what it will do about future medical education. This too needs to be followed carefully.

Historical Perspective

ROSEMARY A. STEVENS, PH.D.

The 1910 Flexner report, to which Dr. Anlyan referred in his presentation, made three points that I would like to challenge because I think they are relevant not only to the history of medicine in the United States but to our discussions as well. First, the report mentioned the right of the state to deal with medical education; second, it referred to the physician as a social instrument; and third, it defined the medical school as a public service corporation.

I would like to suggest, first, that the role of the physician as a social instrument is dead. When Flexner talked in 1910 about the physician as a social instrument, he was talking in a climate of enormous faith in medical research and enormous change through advancements in medical science. The advancement of medical science was seen as a social good. The physician, as an instrument of scientific advance, was a social instrument and, indeed therefore, the reformation, upgrading, and building of the medical schools was automatically seen as being in the public good.

Dr. Anlyan's presentation very nicely portrayed the fact that many of the questions of medical science existing in 1910 were dealt with very successfully. New issues that we face today raise different questions of the relationships between medicine and what used to be called "the social betterment." The physician is only one social instrument, a segment of the system and increasingly an employee. I think that we, like Great Britain, are moving increasingly into a whole spectrum of closed systems as far as physician employment is concerned. The employment market is changing.

My second point concerns Flexner's allusion to the medical school as a public service corporation. History shows that the medical school has been exquisitely sensitive as a public service corporation over the years, but perhaps not in the way that Flexner intended. It has been enormously responsive to outside funding, to outside stimuli, to external influences over the years. Medical schools have entrepreneurial faculties, a fascinating creative blend able to adjust very quickly to outside demands. The medical school has become a public service corporation but with very special characteristics. So much has the medical school become latched into outside influences of various kinds that we also need to consider the growing market in medical education, the relationship between the U.S. schools and the offshore schools, and new markets for medical education.

My third point is that history shows that it is an illusion to assume that there is a proper public function in the role and production of physicians. First, in terms of how many doctors do we need, who is "we"? Is it government? Is it third party? Is it the foundations? Is it the system? There is no one "we" and there never has been.

I am not sure that looking at the medical schools in terms of the numbers of physicians produced is as important as looking at what the constraints are going to be in the medical system in terms of employment practices and the specialty choices of individual physicians. Are we going to see major changes in medicine as there have been in dentistry, where there is a major change in the applicants' pool? Are we going to continue to expect everybody who goes to medical school to practice medicine? Are they going to be locked into it anyway because of the amount of debt they incur in medical school? Are we going to be willing to put up with unemployed physicians? And what are they going to be doing in the American society of the nineties?

Do we have a self-correcting system here in which people decide that going into medicine is really not worth it?

History teaches us a great deal about the complexities of the issue, the difficulty of prediction and, perhaps most of all, that questions of physician supply are, at the root, really questions of power and money.

GMENAC Revisited

ALVIN R. TARLOV, M.D.

I would like to divide my presentation into three parts. First, to review the GMENAC findings and update them; second, to use internal medicine as a paradigm of the dynamics that are taking place in health manpower; and third, to focus a bit on a third compartment which has developed since the GMENAC report and which is increasing in importance.

The GMENAC Findings

The GMENAC charge in 1977 by the Secretary of HEW, Joseph Califano, was to advise the secretary on the need for physician services in the United States and how those needs could best be met in terms of specialty distribution, geographic distribution, and the financing of graduate medical education.

The first question—how many physicians are needed—was by far the most complex and the most difficult to deal with. In the base year of 1978 there were 375,000 full-time equivalent, actively practicing physicians in the United States which was, according to our calculations, somewhat less than the requirement for physician services. GMENAC projected that by 1990 there would be an increase in the supply of physicians to 536,000 and by the year 2000 to 643,000 physicians.

The assumptions made at that time, which drove the supply model, were five: first, the class size in U.S. medical schools; second, similar size in the class of the osteopathic schools; third, the return of foreign medical graduates to the United States for training and practice; fourth, women physicians' productivity; and fifth, retirement assumptions.

Reviewing these in 1985, I think the following conclusions can be reached. First, we were probably a thousand students per class high in estimating medical school class size. Since that has an effect on the entering of physicians for about an eight-year period, the estimate of 643,000 physicians in the year 2000 is probably too high by about 8,000 to 10,000.

Second, the assumptions made in 1978 in regard to the enrollment in osteopathic medicine in 1988 are probably correct—about 1,868 in each class. That enrollment objective was established by the osteopathic schools in order to reach a total osteopath population of about 10 percent of the total practicing physicians in the United States.

The third assumption, having to do with the foreign medical graduate, is still difficult to unravel, but it would appear that our estimate of the entry rate of 4,100 per year of both U.S. citizens and aliens is close to the mark.

Fourth, in regard to women physician productivity, we calculated the total lifetime productivity of female physicians at 78 percent of that of their male counterparts. We were on target in projecting the number of women physicians in practice in 1990 and 2000. No information has appeared in the intervening years to alter that estimate.

Fifth, regarding retirement age, we based our estimate on the experience of the late 1970s. We did recognize that the growing supply of physicians and the increasing malpractice insurance rates and other changes in the value system of our physician population would likely lead to changes in retirement age, particularly stimulated by the development of IRAs and Keogh retirement plans. It is a little too early for us to reassess that assumption.

Based on those five assumptions I believe we are headed for about 630,000 full-time equivalent, actively practicing physicians in the United States in the year 2000.

Now, on the question of requirements for physicians, we had to make a judgment very early on whether to base our modeling on a need-based model or a demand-based model. We elected to use a need-based model that is based on epidemiologic information and that models each medical condition in terms of its prevalence or incidence and multiplies that by the norms of care for that particular condition, whether it requires hospital visits or visits to the doctor's office or to other facilities. We derived the norms of care by taking a careful look at what they were in 1978 and then, using a panel of experts, predicting changes that likely would occur by the year 1990 and the year 2000. After taking the prevalence and multiplying it by the norms of care, the model divides that by physician productivity, assigns certain segments to nonphysician health care providers, and leaves the remainder for the physician. The assumptions in that model and the judgments that had to be made were recognized at that time as being rather risky. Since our charge was specifically heavily weighted toward the requirements for physician services, however, we felt that we had to proceed with that model. The important point is that the model was based on need rather than demand. We concluded, after calculating the supply and the requirements, that the supply of doctors would exceed the requirements in 1990 and even more so in the year 2000.

At that time, in 1978 and 1980, there were two compartments of medicine in practice. The first compartment, which was the larger, was the fee-for-service compartment, which comprised about 95 percent of all practicing physicians and cared for about that percentage of the U.S. population. The second compartment—the federal compartment—had about 18,000 or 19,000 physicians in military service, the Veterans Administration, the Public Health Service, and other federal positions, serving about 3 percent of the U.S. population.

The characteristics of those two compartments were quite different. Physicians in the second compartment were salaried, hired, and paid by the federal government to provide services to those individuals in the employ of or retired from government service. The system lacked elasticity; the precise number of doctors in each specialty was prescribed. In the first compartment, however, there was a great deal of elasticity. Physicians had the liberty to practice where they wished, the fee structure was responsive to the demands of the physicians, and there seemed to be no limit to the absorptive capacity of this compartment to handle newly trained physicians in any number.

Since that time, the data sources have markedly improved. The AMA data file and annual report continue to provide extraordinarily good information and are being refined all the time. The Educational Commission on Foreign Medical Graduates' information is also better now than it was in 1978. The information that Paul Ellwood has been collecting for almost a decade is proving to be extraordinarily useful.

Internal Medicine

Some of the dynamics in the health manpower field are worth looking at, and I am going to use internal medicine as a paradigm. For the past ten years we have been collecting information on internal medicine residency training each year—R-1 through R-5—by U.S. medical graduates, by U.S. citizens who studied abroad, and by alien foreign medical graduates. There continues to be some growth in the number of internal medicine programs: 438 today compared with 432 two years ago. There also continues to be growth in the number of residents entering internal medicine each year: roughly 35 percent of U.S. medical graduates enter their first year of training in internal medicine. There is a rather sharp drop-off of about 18 percent between the first and the second year, which reflects the fact that a great number of future specialists take their first postgraduate year in internal medicine as preparation for their subsequent specialty. Another 20 percent of all the house officers on duty at any moment are individuals who are taking a one-month or three-month rotation on the internal medicine service.

Thus, about 45 percent of the first year of postgraduate training is provided on the internal medicine services, although in the end about 25 or 26 percent of all physicians are internists. This number is expected to continue to grow until 1987 or 1988 because it annually reflects a similar proportion of the graduating class size. Since entering class size did not begin to level off until 1984 or 1985, this number will continue to rise until the graduating class size begins to level.

Another important point is the distribution of U.S. and alien FMGs. Ten years ago 20 percent of the physicians-in-training in internal medicine were graduates of foreign medical schools but almost all of them, 18 out of the 20 percent, were aliens. In the intervening ten years, the growth of the schools in the Caribbean and in Mexico has changed that.

Today alien foreign medical graduates have a predilection to increasing subspecialization while, as yet at least, the USFMG returning to this country for house officer training has in the last five years gone out into practice as a generalist. Today the USFMGS also seem to be increasing in subspecialty training.

When you put all this information together you can see that the number of U.S. medical graduates is continuing to rise. The number of residents also continues to rise, as it will continue to do for another three years. The number of fellows in internal medicine subspecialization also is continuing to rise roughly in proportion to the total number of residents.

If we look at the number of subspecialty fellows in any year and compare it with the number of third year residents in the previous year, we get an indication of how many internists are entering one of the fifteen subspecialty fields. The results of that calculation —which we call the subspecialization rate—show that about 60 percent of all internists have elected to study and ultimately to practice in a subspecialty of internal medicine. In the mid-seventies, the ratio was even higher. It seems to have leveled off in the current academic year.

We have also collected data on the sources of residents' stipends in 1976 and again seven years later, 1983–84. Today more of it is coming from hospital revenues and less from state and federal governments, federal training grants, and research grants. When one calculates residents' stipends and converts the 1976 figure, using the consumer price index, to 1983 dollars, one immediately detects that residents' stipends have actually declined by about 20 percent in real dollars in that seven-year period. We have seen a similar decline of about 10 or 12 percent in fellowship stipends during that same period.

Using our data, we can project into any future year the expected active U.S. internist population. We can also calculate the number of entrants into the practice of medicine and the number of exitors, using such standard actuarial techniques as the death, disability, and retirement rates. The net increase in each year reflects the number of entrants minus the number of exitors.

Since the average duration of medical practice is about thirty-five years, the entry rate into practice for the 1980s, 1990s, and into the year 2000 depends on present and recent rates of entry into medical school plus the entry of FMGs, while the exitor rate reflects the rates of entry into medical school during the fifties and sixties. As a result of that thirty-five-year gap, the number of entrants will exceed the number of exitors until approximately the year 2015. In other words, the system will be in a positive net balance until that time.

The Third Compartment

When the GMENAC study was done the third compartment of medicine in practice—prepaid capitated care—was relatively small. The growth in this compartment for the past decade has been both profound and sustained. With about fifteen million enrollees in 1985 and a 15 percent annual growth rate, that number will double in about five years. There are no signs at the present time to indicate that there either has been or will be a slowdown in the enrollment in HMOs. This introduces a huge change in manpower considerations because this third compartment, like the second compartment, is inelastic and very lean.

In the year 2000 one would expect 127,000 physicians to be employed in the prepaid plans giving roughly 1.1 physician per thousand population, with the physician per thousand people ratio being three times greater in the first compartment. On a world basis, this is a relatively high physician/population ratio although it has been achieved in some of the Western European countries already.

Conclusions

The supply projections made by GMENAC in 1980, based on five important assumptions, receive near-term partial validation in 1985. In the year 2000, there will be 630,000 full-time equivalent, actively practicing physicians yielding a ratio of 233 physicians per 100,000 population.

The rapid growth in prepaid capitated care will enlarge the third compartment to near predominance by the turn of the century. Because the third compartment is fixed relative to the entry rate of physicians per size of population, an exaggerated, disproportionate distribution of physicians will occur. The residual physicians left for the first compartment in the year 2000 will have a physician/population ratio three times greater than in the third compartment, or a ratio of 334 compared with 106 per 100,000 population. For some of the specialized fields, the ratio will become five, ten, or fifteen times greater. Furthermore, the elasticity or the absorptive capacity of the first compartment is coming under sharp constraint.

The need-based model used by GMENAC for estimating the requirement for physicians is now obsolete because it no longer fits the factors that are governing the system. A demand or economic model is more appropriate.

The Physician Surplus: Another View

WILLIAM B. SCHWARTZ, M.D.

Expert opinions on needs are of interest but if you want to estimate a surplus or deficit of physicians it is necessary to know
something about the demand as well as the supply side of the
equation. For this purpose, standard economic forecasting techniques are the best tools we have available. We know there are a
number of factors that influence demand—individual per capita
income, technologic change, the aging of the population, insurance coverage of physicians' services, and the growth of the
population. Historical data can be used to estimate the effect that
changes in each of these factors have on demand, and all of that
can be aggregated to get a projection of future demand. This can
then be assessed in relation to the estimated growth in supply.

Some years ago, soon after the GMENAC report, Frank Sloan of
Vanderbilt and I used this kind of forecasting model to look at
what the physician demand-supply balance would be in 1990 and
our conclusion was that demand would be slightly higher than
supply, a very different conclusion from the need-based estimate
of GMENAC.

As of the end of 1983 the data indicated very much what our
estimate showed: demand had grown by 5 or 7 percent more than
supply, despite the fact that during that four-year period, supply
had grown considerably. At least at the early period of the decade,
this kind of forecasting technique appeared to have been reasonably reliable.

As a baseline for looking toward the year 2000, we did the same
sort of thing, making rather conservative estimates. We assumed,
for example, that there would be no increase in coverage for
physicians' services, and we made a rather conservative estimate of
the growth of individual per capita income. Our demand-based

model suggests that if business were going on as usual and if none of the reimbursement or regulatory changes had occurred, we would anticipate a demand surplus of about 25 or 30 percent, that is, a more rapid growth in demand than in supply. This stands in rather sharp contrast to the GMENAC projection of demand-supply balance.

Now, obviously, a business-as-usual scenario does not apply. The world has changed dramatically and, in 1985, I think we have to look forward to cost containment and regulatory and competitive strategies that will alter the picture from the one that this business-as-usual scenario yields. So, we have done some backing off from that projection. The first backing off we did was to project that there are 30 percent fewer hospital days, that the country as a whole becomes a gigantic HMO in its behavior toward hospitalization, and that we assume a shift in care to the ambulatory sector from the inpatient side. We also assume a 15 percent demand reduction for physicians' services, which would decrease our excess demand to 10 or 15 percent in the year 2000.

The second backoff we made was in relation to technologic change. Technologic change over the past few years has been contributing three to four percentage points in real growth in hospital expenditures. We have backed off and said suppose a third or a half of that is eliminated by cost containment and constriction of available capital. We start with 1985 as the base year and assume that over the period of 1985 to 2000 demand will grow by 15 or 20 percent less in the aggregate than it would have in the absence of capital constraints and various cost containment strategies. If we back off from our estimate by that additional amount, we are down to either a balance point between demand and supply or, more likely, a 5 or 10 percent surplus of physicians relative to demand.

Finally, we made another estimate in which we assumed supply is growing by 10 or 15 percent more than in the GMENAC projection for the 1990 to 2000 period. That could bring our surplus of physicians to a figure of about 15 or 20 percent.

If we take our best point estimate after the backoffs that I have suggested, we come out somewhere between zero—that is, balance —and a 10 percent surplus of physicians, which is not really a very striking change. However, given the uncertainties in these numbers and the time trends we are dealing with, the possibility that the number could be more like a 15 or 20 percent surplus is certainly a real one.

Given that we think there will be probably at least a slight surplus, it is interesting to consider what the beneficial and perverse effects of such a surplus will be. The market is going to equilibrate. A surplus is not permanent. Things happen, and some of these things, from society's point of view, are very good indeed. You can expect a shorter waiting time to get an appointment with a physician; a shorter waiting time in the physician's office until you get to see him or her; and longer visits on the part of the physician with the patient. With PPOs and capitation there will be a drop in expenditures for physician services per visit, so that with fees falling and these time-price changes, the patient is the beneficiary and the physician is the loser. One of the additional advantages is that you do not have to put signs up in small towns asking doctors to come in or to build offices for them; competition helps in distributing physicians as well.

Now, on the side of adverse effects, the main concern is quality of care. As caseload per physician falls, what happens to quality of care? Do we have to think of that as a dimension that the market will not take care of for us but that the government or others have to deal with by specific interventions on entry or residency mix? There are really no good data on caseload impact per doctor.

A recently published study used regression analysis to try to isolate the effect of mortality rate, per se, from those factors that might simply have correlated with it to see what the impact of volume alone was on the excess mortality rate. Using variables such as the geographic location of the hospital, whether it had residents, and so forth, the authors found that, with the exception of open heart surgery, the volume relationship could account for only 0 to 5 percent of the excess mortality.

The second issue has to do with the quality of applicants entering medical school. The ratio of applicants to acceptances is now two to one. That is lower than a decade ago, but higher than the 1.6 to 1.7 applicants per acceptance of the late 1950s and early 1960s. We still have some distance to go in terms of falloff in applications before we reach that level, and whether we should be concerned now about some further modest drop in quality or number of applicants is an open question. No one is complaining that the middle-aged physician of today, who was drawn from the smaller pool of applicants of the early sixties and late fifties, is not doing a competent job.

To summarize, the best point estimate for the year 2000 is probably a slight surplus of physicians. This probably will have societally beneficial effects in terms of cost, waiting time, and diffusion of physicians. A larger surplus is certainly a possibility, but it does not look as if it is going to be huge. Even if this surplus exists, the documentation of the negative effect still remains unclear. We do not know what a 15 or 20 percent surplus will do in terms of quality of care or effect on applicants.

It seems wise to watch the progress in those areas and to begin more systematic studies of individual physicians and how the overall outcomes, not just inpatient mortality rates, are affected by lower volumes. If we see evidence of a deterioration of quality, intervention at that point will certainly be warranted as it will if the quality of our applicants clearly drops very sharply.

Presently there is very little evidence that we should be intervening, at either the federal or the university level, in constraining entry of medical students. We should, however, be alert to the possibility of intervening later. If by chance society resists the kind of draconian cost containment efforts that are being undertaken, it is possible that demand will rise more than projected in my estimates. If we have restricted entry and the demand rises more than expected, we might find ourselves in a situation where we wish we had some of those doctors we did not allow to enter medical school.

Market Forces and Geographic Distribution of Physicians

JOSEPH P. NEWHOUSE, PH.D.

By modifying a rather simple economic model we will be able to understand both what has happened with respect to physician location and what is likely to happen. This model (figure 6) is a little too simple, but it will serve as a starting point and yield some testable implications that will prove out. The top row of figure 6 illustrates a line that can be thought of as a highway with three towns on it; the towns have populations of five thousand, ten thousand, and thirty thousand. I am going to make some simplified assumptions. First, nobody lives outside these towns. Second, the average demand per person in each of these towns is the same. Third, each of the towns is equally attractive to live in to physicians. I am also going to make behavioral assumptions: first, that physicians locate in a way that maximizes the demand for their services and, second, that people who have to travel for care demand less of it.

Now under those assumptions the first doctor into this little

Figure 6. Physician Diffusion as Supply Grows: Towns of 5,000, 10,000, and 30,000 Population.

Number of physicians of a given specialty in towns with populations of:			Total number of physicians
5,000	10,000	30,000	
0	0	1	1
0	0	2	2
0	1	3	4
1	2	6	9
2	4	12	18

world of three towns (top row) goes to the town of thirty thousand. If he went to one of the other two towns, the people in the town of thirty thousand would have to travel and they would demand less of him than if he went to the town of thirty thousand.

The second doctor (second row) also goes to the town of thirty thousand. Only when we have four doctors (third row) does a first doctor appear in the town of ten thousand. Finally, when we get up to nine doctors (fourth row) there is a doctor out in the town of five thousand. Thereafter as the number of doctors grows the towns gain doctors proportionately in this simple model.

There are three testable implications that I want to draw from this little model. The first is that for any given number of doctors there is a critical town size; towns above that size have a doctor and towns below it do not. For example, in figure 6 the critical town size is between five and ten thousand when we have four doctors. Critical town size falls as the number of doctors increases so as we increase the number of doctors beyond nine the critical town size decreases below five thousand.

Second, if we look at figure 6 as different specialties instead of one specialty growing over time, and if the different specialties do not compete with each other, we will find, for example, the general surgeons out in smaller towns and the neurosurgeons in larger towns.

Finally, if we regard this model as concerning one specialty that grows through time, smaller towns are going to gain physicians at a proportionately faster rate. For example, if we combine the towns of five and ten thousand populations and look at the change between four doctors and nine doctors, we would go from one doctor in those two towns to three doctors, a tripling, whereas in the town of thirty thousand we would only increase from three to six, or a doubling.

This simple model was somewhat discredited in the late 1960s and 1970s, I think wrongly. These are the facts on which it was discredited. First, there is the well-known disparity in metropolitan and nonmetropolitan physician ratios, but this is not in and of itself inconsistent with the model. This disparity disturbed many people in terms of the access of nonmetropolitan people to physicians. Particularly in the late sixties, we were producing a lot more doctors, and almost all of them were going to metropolitan areas. Even in the seventies, when this disparity evened up and then disappeared, physician numbers were still growing a little bit faster in the metropolitan areas.

Using the AMA master data file in 1970 and 1979 we looked at towns in twenty-three rural states that have a population of more than 2,500. Forty percent of towns of five to ten thousand had an internist in 1970 and that had grown to 52 percent in 1979. The first implication is that there is a critical town size: towns above it have a physician, towns below it do not. That is not exactly observed, however, and the reason it is not is because my simplifying assumptions are not exactly correct: there *are* populations outside towns; towns are *not* equally attractive to physicians to locate in; and the demand per person in different towns is *not* the same. What that means is that there is a tendency for larger towns to have a physician of a given type. Another implication is that the larger specialties will be further out in the smaller communities, but that the smaller towns are less likely to have certain subspecialists.

Everything that I have said up until now has been premised on the notion that the various specialties do not compete with each other, but in fact they do and this has two kinds of consequences. First, consider the competition between an internist and a general practitioner located along a highway with the population uniformly distributed along this highway. If the population cannot tell the difference between the two physicians or if they do not care about the difference and if physicians who are referring also do not care about the difference, then I would draw a line about halfway down the highway and people on one side of the line would go to the internist while the people on the other side of the line would go to the general practitioner. If, however, the internist faces more demand, then I would draw the line closer to the general practitioner and the internist would get a larger share of the population. The implication of this is that where the internist goes head-to-head against the general practitioner in a city and tends to win that competition, the general practitioner is going to be more willing to go to a smaller town than the internist. The same would be true if the board-certified physician tends to win against the noncertified physician, or if the USMG tends to win against the FMG.

There is a second phenomenon that exists with this interspecialty competition: specialists such as internists and pediatricians produce some services that general practitioners either do not produce at all or tend not to produce. The internist with unique services is like that first specialist into the town of five thousand, ten thousand, and thirty thousand: he goes into the larger town but once he is there he also produces basic services. Seeing the internist in the larger town, the general practitioner tends to go toward the smaller town.

The result of most of these phenomena is that small towns tend to have almost all general practitioners. In towns with fewer than 25,000 people, a majority of the physicians are general practitioners. Even in cities with 25,000 to 50,000 population, a near majority of the physicians are general practitioners. In the large metropolitan areas, however, only around 20 percent of the physicians are general practitioners.

During the sixties and seventies there was, of course, a decline in the number of general practitioners. The family practice programs came into being in the seventies but they did not produce enough graduates in the seventies to offset the decline of the general practitioner, although they started to by the 1980s. The specialties, meanwhile, were growing quite rapidly in the 1970s and growth is clearly continuing in the 1980s. Indeed all specialties are going to grow in the 1980s.

The drastic decrease in the number of general practitioners being produced greatly affected the small town physician supply and we saw the beginning of advertising for physicians. The critical town size for the specialist was falling, but it was not low enough to compensate for the decline in the number of general and family practitioners.

Around 20 percent or so of the population does not live in towns of 25,000 or more. In fact, most of those people do not live in towns at all. The question is, How far do those people have to travel to reach the nearest physician of a given kind? In 1979, 70 to 80 percent of the rural population was within roughly half an hour of an internist. Almost half the population in 1979 was within thirty straight line miles of a neurosurgeon.

One of the problems that we run into when we look at the question of medical care for metropolitan versus nonmetropolitan residents is the assumption that all the nonmetropolitan residents get their care from nonmetropolitan physicians. For some of them, however, the closest physician is in a metropolitan area. When looking at physician/population ratios, those people need to be taken out of the denominator of the nonmetropolitan ratio and moved over to the metropolitan ratio. That does not much affect the metropolitan ratio but it does affect the nonmetropolitan ratio.

The important point is that physicians do seem to choose their location in accordance with standard economic models. As all specialties increase in numbers in the 1980s and 1990s, we can expect the critical town size to fall still further and the numbers of physicians in the rural areas to increase still further.

Correcting "Surpluses" and "Shortages" in Medical Specialties

I. The Surgeons
C. ROLLINS HANLON, M.D.

Fifteen years ago in the cutting edge of developing physicians—in the residency area—the surgeons constituted slightly over 40 percent of all residencies whereas primary care physicians—not including obstetrics-gynecology—constituted 25 percent of all the residencies. In 1983–84, the figure for surgeons is down to 28 percent of all residencies, whereas for primary care it has risen to almost 43 percent. We have seen an inversion of the manpower situation of fifteen years ago.

When the prophets on manpower have so obviously missed the mark thus far, why are we to assume that their projections will be any more accurate this time around? We all know that it takes five years or more before it is obvious that events have overrun forecasts in the most predictable way; no one seems capable of foretelling the future in manpower. The historical landscape is littered with the burned out reports of eminent commissions and leaders of American medicine who embarked on fortune telling and succeeded only in demonstrating that their crystal ball had a defect in its lattice structure.

What can an international organization of some 55,000 surgeons do about surpluses and shortages? What we should do first is to change what Paul Rogers has called the public perception. Changing that perception of the public at large—including the media, academic and other planners, the various segments of local and federal government, the insurance industry, the business community whether directly involved or indirectly related to health, and the organized patients such as the 18 million individuals in the American Association of Retired Persons and other consumer groups—is a formidable and probably an impossible task, particularly if we are not certain whether we can project a surplus or a shortage.

Where are the possible points of influence by the American College of Surgeons? First, we can analyze and in some instances collect data on surgical services, both operative and nonoperative. We can attempt to determine whether these services are being provided by real surgeons, by surgical pretenders among physicians, or by nonphysicians. We can track the number and activities of surgical residents, the growing edge of surgical manpower resources.

The College has always had a strong interest in and a substantial influence on the quality of surgical education. For the past several years, we have resumed the maintenance of accurate data about individuals in the surgical residency system, placing it in context with other databases of the Association of American Medical Colleges, the AMA, the National Resident Matching Program (NRMP), and the surgical specialty societies themselves. Not only do we know accurately where these young men and women are but we have individual reports from some 8,000 of them about what they are doing in the way of caseload and activity.

The ACS has representatives on various boards and on the Residency Review Committees where, with due regard for quality, fairness, and the brooding presence of the Federal Trade Commission, a monitoring effect may be exerted on surgical quality, with possible secondary effects on the numbers of programs and then on the total number of individuals who emerge from surgical graduate medical education. This is a very sensitive area; if the residency review committees and the boards begin to deliberately exert surgical birth control on those programs, I think they run a great risk of being under the gun of a Federal Trade Commission summons.

Surgical program directors are concluding on their own that it is desirable to restrict the number of physicians. They may carry out this restriction either by instituting a pyramidal system—under which individuals are displaced from the pyramid at the second, third, or some higher level—or by truncating it deliberately from the outside by nonfunding of physicians at some arbitrary level. Those of us who are convinced that you cannot educate a surgeon adequately in, say, three years after medical school, find the rigid prescription of arbitrary time intervals more offensive than cutting down on the number of individuals allowed into the program. On the one hand, we end up with a reasonable number of inadequately educated surgeons—I am not saying "trained" surgeons although training is a component there; on the other hand, we have an inadequate number of reasonably well educated surgeons. In each instance, the decision will be based on a preconception about the proper proportion of various specialists in a presumed ideal mix that is established by something akin to a need-based formula. These formulas may not last, however. They are strongly influenced by the backgrounds and prejudices of those who are involved in their construction.

I come back to the starting point of the American College of Surgeons, which is quality, and our underlying conviction that education to provide the highest quality of surgical care in every individual who comes before us will ultimately result in better care for the patient. While this does not absolutely prove that there is a direct relationship between high quality of education and delivery of better care, I believe quite strongly that that *is* the case.

Should we, if we have the influence and the chance, cut down on the number of surgeons or press for expansion? I think we will leave that question unanswered.

II. The Physicians
ROBERT H. MOSER, M.D.

The position of both Colleges is quite similar. We really do not have any direct impact on the manpower situation. We are, of course, vitally interested in the subject, and we do participate in such things as the residency review committee, and we have an informal relationship with our board, the American Board of Internal Medicine.

I think it goes without saying that we have primed the pump a little too effectively. If we were to shut down all the medical schools tomorrow, we would still apparently have an overall surplus of doctors by the year 2000. I stress the word "overall." In my mind, by far the larger issue is the geographical, specialty, and subspecialty distribution. There may well be too many psychiatrists in Beverly Hills. There may well be too many cardiologists in Boston. But are there enough psychiatrists in El Centro and are there enough cardiologists in Laramie? If not, how do we equilibrate the situation and get them to switch around? What impact will telecommunications—the capability to have consultation via computer—and the expanding new technologies have on rural practices and the distribution of specialists and subspecialists across the country?

What impact will the growth of other health care practitioners have on physician manpower? All of these factors are most difficult to assess.

From the aspect of internal medicine, the subject has been discussed at great length. It is the subject of a major position paper and has been bandied about at the Federated Council of Internal Medicine. At the moment we have no solutions, but there are some points worthy of discussion. There are still about 35 or 36 percent of young people out of the 16,000 annual medical school graduates who go into internal medicine as PG-1s. About 61 percent of these physicians then go into the subspecialties, leaving about 39 percent who go into primary care internal medicine. We have a feeling that this number might be inadequate for the future.

There are several mechanisms whereby we can try to slow down the flow of personnel. First, what can the American Board of Internal Medicine do? As with the surgical board, they could arbitrarily increase the cut-off score for certification or they could make exams much tougher. They could make it more difficult to get a certificate of special competence; they could simply produce fewer certificates both in internal medicine and in its subspecialties; or they could simply increase the time between graduation from medical school and the time when one can sit for the ABIM. Now one can sit for the board three years out of medical school and take the exam for the certificate of special competence within another two years. It can all be compressed to a total of four years. Lengthening this period of time would certainly slow down the pipeline. We are all pretty much opposed in principle to arbitrarily increasing the flunk rate as a means of control. However, there are many of us who think that the time frame could be lengthened, both for ABIM and for a certificate of special competence certification.

Second, what about the RRCIM? A residency review committee could certainly set tougher standards for internal medicine residency programs. Now that all the subspecialty programs are coming under our purview, we could do the same for them with the blessing of the Accreditation Council on Graduate Medical Education (ACGME). Both the RRCIM and the ABIM have refused to become vehicles for the solution of this vexing social and economic problem, and I endorse that and so does our College.

The RRCIM could tighten the screws. They could put perhaps 30 percent of the marginal programs that they see on probation if they decided to get a great deal tougher. In addition, the ACGME can arbitrarily say that they will not accept individuals for post-graduate medical education unless they come from LCME medical schools, a very difficult political decision from many aspects. I am inclined to agree with the stance of the ABIM and the RRC that they cannot afford to become politicized, not only from the aspect of conflict with the FTC but also because they still stand as major bastions of excellence.

Third, what could program directors do? Those in the Association of Professors of Medicine, those in the Association of Program Directors in Internal Medicine, and those who run subspecialty fellowships could tighten the screws and decrease the number of available slots in their individual programs. But can you expect individual program directors to act either positively or negatively in response to a social need? They have never done this before. They have mandated the number of participants in their programs on the basis of resources, patient needs, equipment, and faculty, and they have never yielded to the necessity to respond to social responsibility. I am not sure they could if they had to, unless driven by some external force.

Although there has been some cutback in some programs, there is also an acceleration. In 1984, we had 1,518 individual sub-specialty programs in internal medicine; in 1985 it is up to 1,557. Rather than decreasing, it has increased by some thirty-nine programs. There are a few less cardiology programs and a few more oncology programs, but basically there has been only a little change. Predictably, however, there will be a change: there will be a cutback.

Indeed, there will be a major change in many programs if the Part B Medicare reimbursement for direct resident pay actually comes to pass, and most of us think that will happen. Many programs will be obliged either to cut back or to become very creative in seeking new sources of funding for graduate medical education.

In addition, the personnel flow is sensitive to other sources of federal and state funding. The flow of primary care residents in family practice, internal medicine, and pediatrics was expanded through specific federal granting programs. We were concerned about that because it possibly served to the detriment of other residency programs. It is conceivable that in the new world the control could become even more exquisite, with selective federal or even state funding of specific undersubscribed subspecialties under payback provisions that would oblige recipients of this largesse to serve where needed for specified periods, somewhat analogous to the National Health Service Corps. This possibly could succeed because the need is greater. This mechanism also has precedent in the private sector. Some communities lacking a physician have sponsored young people all the way through medical school and residency training just to ensure that they will have a physician in the community. The same mechanism will also occur in industry and other organizations seeking to employ physicians with specific specialty and subspecialty skills.

There may be a time when we will accept foreign medical graduates with the specific intent that they be trained here and then returned to their country. It may well be that the State Department could use this as a foreign aid program. Wouldn't it be helpful if we could continue to expand residencies and provide a supply of well-trained individuals for countries that needed them?

A final mechanism that we have heard about would be through the market place, as some equilibration occurs through reimbursement revision and policy. Perhaps there will be fewer ophthalmology or cardiovascular aspirants as financial incentives decline. This alone might increase the attractiveness of primary care careers.

Thus, there are many factors with the potential for influencing the numbers, both in absolute terms and with respect to geographical and subspecialty applicants. At the American College of Physicians, we will continue to monitor the physician supply while ensuring that the high quality of internal medicine in this country will continue.

Life-style Choices and Evolving Practice Patterns

BRITAIN NICHOLSON, M.D.

There is really no question that we are in the midst of a very dramatic change regarding physician life-styles and practice patterns. Physicians are restructuring their practices to allow greater flexibility and more predictable hours; residents are asking for more personal time, primarily in the forms of maternity and paternity leaves; and medical students are electing careers that allow for more time for personal relationships, balanced with sufficient secure salaries to allow them to pay back ever-mounting and staggering educational debts. What this means for the late eighties and the nineties is really a trend toward shift work—salaried positions with predictable hours in institutional settings—or else the more procedure-oriented subspecialty careers that for now will give a much higher reimbursement and much higher income prediction than the more primary care-oriented subspecialties.

At the risk of being too simplistic and sounding like a fundamentalist minister, I think that the two forces responsible for this evolution are women and money. It would be a mistake to assume that this is just a women's issue. This issue really affects men and women equally, but there is no question that the relatively recent entry of women into working and professional roles has influenced the current trends we perceive. Female physicians have increased dramatically in number in the past decade. In 1983 women comprised 32 percent of all medical students nationally and 25 percent of all residents. Thirty-three percent of these women were married and 10 percent were engaged at the time of graduation. These women are graduating in their mid to late twenties and anticipating residency and career building during the height of their childbearing years, and this necessitates a greater flexibility in life-style and in practice pattern.

The 1984 AMA report on maternity leave for residents found that 26 percent of female residents have children and 63 percent of practicing female physicians have children. The resident number is probably a low estimate given that the pool of respondents was generally an older group of women who were active in the AMA. Nevertheless, 45 percent of women with children had their first child during their training and 27 percent of women had at least two children during their training.

At the time of this survey, four-fifths of women reportedly did not adjust their schedules before or after delivery and only took a two- to eight-week maternity leave, tending toward the two-week side, and I submit that this is just plain unhealthy. However, this survey probably does not reflect the informal ways in which women shave off hours here and there to fulfill their responsibilities. As life-style choices are more explicitly discussed, part-time roles will definitely become more explicitly defined.

A second important fact is the increasing number of married male residents and medical students. In 1983, 41 percent of graduating male medical students were married and 9 percent were engaged. This is in bold contradistinction to the pattern of earlier years when bachelor house officers virtually lived in hospitals. Because of the increase of women in the work place, many of these marriages are dual-career marriages. Eleven percent of these men are married to women with doctorate level education and 47 percent of the women are married to men with doctorate level education. As dual-career families, many of these graduating students are more explicitly including family concerns in their career decisions.

At Harvard Medical School, a nine-week workshop is offered to students on the impact of a demanding medical career on personal relationships. It is always filled with its quota of twenty students, often all couples. The major concerns of these couples are when to get married, when to have children, and what will be the institutional reaction to maternity leave or schedule adjustments for the family. They express concern about how they can meet the expectations at work of themselves, their peers, their mentors, and their patients and, on a very personal level, their societal expectations for themselves as spouses and parents. One of the faculty leaders of this course has the impression that students who are married or plan to be married are increasingly openly rejecting careers that do not allow flexibility, such as the subspecialty-oriented surgical practices or solo or small-group primary care practices.

Many who desire academic careers fear that they cannot compete as they face the traditional triple threat in teaching, patient care, and research as well as maintaining a healthy family life. Those who choose a generalist's role choose an institutional or large-group setting with salary, controlled hours, and infrequent on-call demands. If they anticipate a twenty-five year period of children's expenses, culminating in the backbreaker—college —they want to earn enough money while they are working to manage these expenses. Money as defined by educational debt, income, and future reimbursement policies are all having their effect.

Though educational debt is rising, it currently does not emerge as a strong predictor of specialty choice or practice setting. In fact, in a recent survey carried out by the AAMC for the Department of Health and Human Services (HHS), the amount of debt as a predictor of career choice—the career choice being high pay versus low pay—ranked seventh. The two top predictors turned out to be sex and whether you attended a public or a private medical school.

Future reimbursement policies will also have some effect on career choice. The procedure-oriented subspecialties are currently very attractive, primarily for their high income. The eighties and nineties will see increasing numbers of men and women choosing, first, shift work because of flexible hours; second, large-group or institutional settings; and third, subspecialties with reimbursement procedures.

I think there will be a decreasing number of physicians choosing entrepreneurial activities like solo practice, because of its financial risk and inflexibility. This will culminate in a continuing decrease of those individuals going into primary care or generalist roles.

Market Influences of FMGS

SAMUEL P. ASPER, M.D.

Twenty-five years ago our nation addressed the problem of a physician shortage by fostering both development of new schools of medicine and enlarged enrollment of students in existing schools. To date these advances have resulted in the production of about 60,000 more physicians than would have graduated under former conditions. Concomitantly, our government permitted, and to some extent encouraged, the immigration, naturalization, and licensure of qualified alien physicians, who today number about 100,000.

This latter approach to solving our health manpower needs was abetted by strong market forces, as alien physicians saw opportunities for job and financial security in the United States. By the mid-seventies the number of physicians from abroad achieving licensure annually nearly equaled that of graduates of U.S. schools, and suddenly the portent of a physician surplus was envisioned. Our Congress, in writing Public Law 94-484 in 1976, stated: "There is no longer an insufficient number of physicians and surgeons in the United States" and discontinued the granting of immigration preference to alien doctors. A decrease in immigration followed. During the past decade, however, many more U.S. citizens began the study of medicine abroad than formerly, and a steady annual increase in the number of U.S. citizen FMGS obtaining licensure ensued.

The AMA Division of Survey and Data Resources[1] indicates that in 1983, of 519,545 physicians in the United States, 112,005 were FMGS. Of these, 80,044 were aliens or former aliens and 31,961 were U.S. citizen FMGS. Thus, FMGS, with a 22 percent repre-

---

1 AMA Physician Masterfile, Data Release Services, Division of Survey and Data Resources (Chicago: American Medical Association, 1985).

sentation, clearly influence the U.S. professional marketplace. Some complain the market is disturbed, others believe it is benefitted, but all agree that the role of FMGS is significant and that new issues result when one in every five physicians among us attains professional status by a route not familiar to most of us.

The tracking of FMGS in the marketplace is not an easy task. The Immigration and Naturalization Service has discontinued its valuable practice of collecting data on immigrant physicians. There is no central clearinghouse on the total number of exchange visitors, as approximately 250 different organizations can and do sponsor them. Also difficult to track are USFMGS. Moreover, little is known about the hundreds of FMGS who never achieve ECFMG certification and are denied entry into graduate clinical training; as unlicensed physicians, do they participate in paramedical activities?

In this presentation I shall highlight briefly some market influences of foreign medical graduates. Equally important to note, however, is the fact that the market also influences foreign medical graduates; one perspective requires the other. Four areas will be covered: foreign medical graduates in graduate medical education, medical practice, academe, and international medicine.

In graduate education it is predicted that economic and other factors in hospitals may soon force a reduction in the number of residencies. To date, however, no decrease has occurred, but there are striking changes in the number of alien and USFMGS entering residencies. Although the number of applications from alien physicians is increasing sharply, the percentage of those obtaining positions is decreasing; in contrast, the number of USFMGS is steadily increasing. It appears that program directors increasingly are giving preference to USFMGS for appointment to residencies, despite the oft-voiced criticism of the educational programs at the offshore medical schools. In 1983 the 13,221 FMGS in residency programs comprised 18.4 percent of the total number of residents. Of the 13,221, 6,231 were alien FMGS and 6,990 were USFMGS.[2]

Recent studies have confirmed that FMGS enter residencies that are less attractive to graduates of U.S. schools, chiefly physical medicine, anesthesiology, pathology, therapeutic radiology, nuclear medicine, and psychiatry. Accordingly, FMGS assist these underserved specialties.

2   Data from *Physician Characteristics and Distribution in the U.S., 1983 Edition* (Chicago: American Medical Association, Division of Survey and Data Resources, 1984).

In the practice of medicine alien FMGS also fill underserved regional and specialty areas. They practice among the urban poor, such as in some of the boroughs of New York City, and in sparsely populated rural areas, such as in West Virginia. Many anecdotal reports describe their beneficial roles. The USFMGS, however, appear to follow practice patterns of graduates of U.S. schools. Moreover, there is some evidence that alien FMGS, after working several years in underserved areas, move to the traditional patterns followed by U.S. physicians.

The extent to which alien FMGS participate in academe may come as a surprise, for new data from the AAMC show that 15.7 percent of all full-time positions in medical schools are held by alien FMGS.[3] The distribution by rank shows that 27.6 percent are professors, 26.2 percent are associate professors, 35.7 percent are assistant professors, 9.3 percent are instructors and below, and the remainder are in the category of "other." The explanation for significant participation of alien FMGS in academe is, I believe, that those FMGS who perform well in residency posts are subsequently retained by departmental chairmen for teaching, patient care, and research positions.

Few data are available on the extent of FMG participation in research. AAMC faculty roster data show that 69 percent of full-time FMG faculty are involved in research on at least a part-time basis. Among appointees to the staff of the National Institutes of Health, 50 percent are foreign nationals who studied medical science abroad. My unsubstantiated opinion is that USFMGS in full-time research are few and that the number of alien physicians is far greater than is generally appreciated.

An examination of the December 1984 issue of the *Journal of Clinical Endocrinology and Metabolism* provided informative data on the research activities of FMGS. Of thirty-four scientific articles, twenty came from medical centers in the United States and fourteen from abroad. Of ninety-one contributing authors and coauthors to the twenty papers from U.S. medical centers, thirteen (15 percent) were alien physicians holding ECFMG certification.

Not to be overlooked is the influence of FMGS in the international, professional, and economic marketplace. Alien foreign medical graduates, following graduate study in the United States, benefit our economy through their purchase of medical journals and texts,

3 *AAMC Faculty Roster System* (Washington, D.C.: Association of American Medical Colleges, 1985).

medical equipment, and pharmaceuticals. Moreover, many physicians who have never studied in the United States hold American medicine in high regard. For example, ECFMG certification is proudly displayed as evidence of meeting a U.S. standard, and qualifying for election to membership in one of our medical specialty societies is a high honor. Also, as mentioned, fourteen, or 40 percent, of the papers in the December 1984 issue of the *Journal of Clinical Endocrinology and Metabolism* came from abroad, showing, among other things, the interest of foreign investigators in publishing in a U.S. journal as well as the acceptability of their research for publication.

Conversely, Americans studying medicine at proprietary medical schools abroad have a significant effect on the economy of the nations in which these schools are located, especially the smaller nations in the Caribbean. Tuition at these offshore schools can be as high as $15,000 annually, and the estimates of the number of Americans enrolled in these schools range from 8,000 to 15,000.

Fluctuations in the FMG marketplace characterize events of the past twenty-five years. Educational opportunity, work availability, and job security are the major contributing factors that determine entry of both foreign national physicians on either temporary or permanent status in the United States and Americans studying medicine abroad who seek to enter practice upon their return. Legislation also has produced fluctuations, from former free entry of qualified alien physicians to controlled entry at present, to proposed regulations that would limit the number of residencies in U.S. medical centers to graduates of LCME-accredited schools.

This is indeed an important moment to reassess our role in international medicine, to evaluate the impact on our health care system of increasing numbers of returning Americans who have studied medicine abroad, and to reconsider our responsibility to global medicine. To the greatest extent possible, we must wisely attempt to create and guide market forces so that our superb educational and research system becomes an effective tool in international diplomacy and goodwill.

Methodological Problems in Assessing Physician Demand, Need, and Supply: Policy Implications

UWE E. REINHARDT, PH.D.

The question that rises in my mind is why are we so concerned about physician manpower in general? I will focus on methodological issues in health manpower forecasting, which is a can of worms itself. What one is asked to do in a manpower forecast is begin with a population which begets the physicians and also begets the clients of the physician—the patients. Right here one has a problem. First of all, one must know about the immigration of physicians, which is a political issue; then one needs occupational choice models, not only to know how many people in the potential pool choose to become physicians, but also their specialty choices.

There are many ways to intervene in manpower planning. One could, for example, raise tuition. Assume that every medical student would have to borrow $25,000 at the beginning of the four medical school undergraduate years. Then charge 10 percent interest on the money with no repayment during the residency. In the ninth year out, they would begin to amortize that debt, which, by that time, would be $200,000. While that seems like a big number, in fact it is not if you amortize it over twenty years at 10 percent, like a mortgage. The annual payment is then about 10 percent of a physician's gross income. That is one way one might influence the supply of physicians.

On the demand side, we have epidemiological models that give us morbidity patterns. The translation of a morbidity pattern into demand for services is quite complicated and may, in fact, depend on how many physicians there are. At least some of us believe that there is a potential on the part of the physicians to manipulate demand. Given that you have a demand for services and a supply of physicians and some model that translates human bodies into output of services, what we would really like to know is are the supply and demand of medical services in balance? The supply of physicians depends on the number of living physicians multiplied by the number of those who are professionally active, which depends, for example, on retirement patterns and on how often physicians drop out during childbearing years. This is multiplied by the number of physicians who give patient care. The resulting sum is the supply side of the forecasting equation (figure 7).

On the demand side you need a population forecast, even though they are not always accurate. If you know the number of services needed, you divide that by the number of services delivered per physician to get the number of physicians needed. This productivity parameter depends on hourly productivity times number of hours worked per week times number of weeks worked per year. All of these factors can and do vary. According to AMA data, the number of hours physicians work has decreased over time.

To show you also the tenuousness of the link between manpower and services, in the seventies in New England there was a population/physician ratio of $161:1$, in the East South Central states of only $95:1$. Despite this disparity, visits per doctor were roughly

Figure 7. A Simple Forecasting Equation for Physician Manpower.

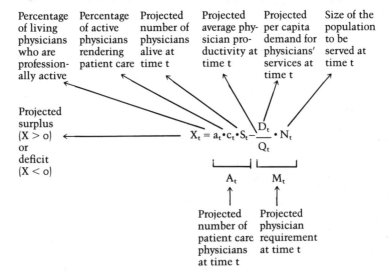

Where Q = hourly productivity × hours/week × weeks/years

Table 1. Average Number of Office Visits per Year by Gender of
Physician: Internal Medicine, United States, 1981.

Variable	Male N = 549	Female N = 46	Female Male
Office visits/hour	2.451	1.99	0.81
Hours per week devoted to office visits	27.18	25.19	0.92
No. of weeks in practice year (1981)	46.43	43.15	0.92
Estimated office visits/year	3092	2163	0.70

Calculated as office visits/hour × office hours/week × weeks/year
Source: Data provided by the American Medical Association.

Table 2. Differentials in Workload of Men and Women Physicians in
Private Practice: France, 1981.

Specialty and age	Patient billings /year		Visits & consultations /year	
	Men	Women	Men	Women
General practice	Frs.	Frs.		
Age 35 or less	262,000	138,000	3,863	1,919
35 to 44 years	358,000	187,000	5,280	2,412
45 to 54 years	349,000	183,000	5,105	2,340
55 to 64 years	303,000	171,000	4,234	2,099
65 years or older	201,000	113,000	2,818	1,448
All general practitioners	305,000	157,000	4,452	2,087

Source: Adapted from CREDOC (1984), table 46, p. 93.

the same in all regions; that is, physicians made up for shortages
in their numbers by seeing patients at a faster clip. To what extent
that affected quality I do not know, but some of this was accomplished by having more aides per physician and also by physicians
being more frequently in a group. In New England physicians were
not often in group practices while in the South they were in group
practices and they had more substitute personnel. You can trade
off different types of manpower for physicians.

The number of women physicians in the supply is increasing. Table 1 shows the average number of patients per office hour for female physicians and for male physicians. Female physicians see roughly 70 percent as many patients in the office per hour as male physicians. Data from 1981 show that women doctors work fewer hours each week and fewer weeks per year. The situation is even worse in France (table 2). The average woman physician in France had 2,087 office visits and consultations in 1981 while male physicians had 4,452. Male French physicians billed an average of 305,000 francs per year while women physicians billed 157,000 francs.

Figure 8 is a somewhat irreverent graph that defines the physician surplus in economic terms. Total dollars expended on physician services per year in a society is on the abscissa and the number of doctors is on the ordinate. If doctors want to realize a certain income and the number of doctors is increasing, more money must be made available to them to meet their desire; that is line A

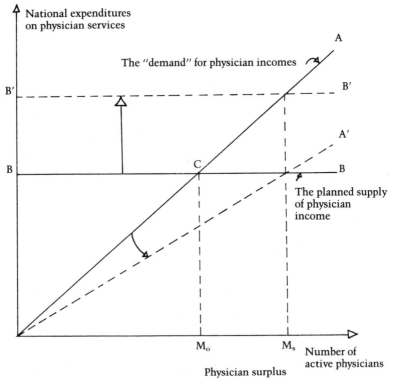

Figure 8. An Economic Definition of a Physician Surplus.

in the figure. Line B is the supply of physician income, the dollars we are willing to make available, around $70 billion now. To an economist, the proper supply of physicians is point C where the two meet, where we are willing to supply what the doctors want.

If you have a surplus of physicians, you have three options. One is to cut back the surplus. While this is a tempting approach, economists would certainly not like it and it raises constitutional issues. Why should you single out some people and say they cannot participate in this game? An alternative option is to lower physician income from A to A', which society is happy to provide to meet the excess supply. The third option, which is probably the one physicians would prefer, is to raise expenditures from B to B' and give them their usual and customary income at that higher level.

If I were asked to give some advice, I would say first of all do not expect too much from forecasting models. Second, you can use these models intelligently by doing sensitivity analyses, by asking "what if?" questions: What is the worst that could happen? What is the most likely? Before intervening on the supply side, I think it would be good to wait and see if the market somehow sorts the problem out. We should perhaps have more faith in the market.

Discussion

DR. PAUL M. ELLWOOD, JR.: We have been collecting data in Los Angeles that tend to support Dr. Tarlov's predictions for the effect of the third compartment—prepaid medical care—not in the year 2000 but right now. At the present time Los Angeles has 7,700,000 people and it has almost 20,000 physicians, giving a physician/population ratio of about 2.6 per thousand. GMENAC forecasts 2.4 per thousand by the year 2000, so there are slightly more physicians per thousand people already in Los Angeles than will be true of the country as a whole in the year 2000.

The HMO enrollment in group practice plans in Los Angeles is now 2,869,000, which exceeds somewhat the figures that Dr. Tarlov used for the year 2000. Incidentally, HMO growth in Los Angeles has slowed from what is now a national average of 21.8 percent per year to about 11 percent per year. If we use the exponential growth curve logic, by the year 1992, 76 percent of the population of the Los Angeles area will be in HMOs.

Kaiser, the dominant HMO in this marketplace, uses about one doctor for every eight hundred people. In Los Angeles, 3,586 physicians are involved in HMO plans where the physician/population ratio is going to be 1:800. Physicians outside the HMOs number about 16,370, and each of these has about 299 prospective patients; of course this varies by specialty.

What is particularly interesting about this situation is its impact on those who are competing with HMOs. In California the number of doctor visits per patient is the lowest in the United States, while the fees of physicians are the highest in the country and the rate of growth of physician income has exceeded the rate of the consumer price index. As a result, the insurance companies that support the activity of non-HMO physicians in California are in serious trouble because they are so much more costly than the HMOs with which they are competing. So we have the phenomenon of a rising supply of physicians accelerating the rate of the development of medical care firms that must rely on even fewer physicians to make it. If we project Dr. Tarlov's numbers out at a few years, we end up with a revised GMENAC report that shows an oversupply of physicians unable to find patients to take care of.

DR. RICHARD S. WILBUR: There is a good bit of evidence already that the number of hours physicians work is being reduced. I am curious about the trends in number of hours worked in the third compartment—the HMOS—particularly in view of their desire to lure physicians who are interested in having more shift work and especially interested in working fewer hours in the delivery of care.

To look at the third compartment and say that the present ratio of physicians to patients is the one that will exist when a vast majority of patients are within HMOs overlooks the fact that the HMO systematically chooses the healthy people. They do this not just because they want to make more money, but because they are the easiest people for the HMOs to enroll since they seek their patients in larger corporations. It is necessary to look at demographics of the patients in HMOs to make sure that Dr. Ellwood's latest figures really reflect the ratio of physicians to patients that will occur when significant numbers of both the indigent and the aged are in HMOs.

When we use models for the geographic distribution of physicians that are based on the fact that every physician is a solo practitioner, I think we have left the realm of future reality. That is a little like projecting clothing supplies by the number of tailors in the United States, or the delivery of food by the number of Mom and Pop grocery stores, or the amount of gasoline by the number of service stations. All of these have declined sharply over the last few years, while the supply of clothing, food, and gas has increased tremendously.

People no longer go to a local store from rural America; they drive to Sears or the discount stores and they load up for the week. That is how medical care will be delivered: more and more by group practices centered in and around the hospitals or other large facilities. Much of the concern about getting a physician at every crossroad is diametrically opposed to the way our society is moving.

PROFESSOR ELI GINZBERG: In New York City we are now spending about 14 percent of city income on medical care. We have very high ratios of physicians to patients—they have in fact already met Dr. Tarlov's estimates for the year 2000—yet we have lots of people in several of our boroughs who cannot get near a physician when they need one. New York City has all the complexities today that you worry about in the year 2000. This is another way of saying that all efforts at national calculations are not very relevant when you introduce the class, race, and other distributional factors that are very important.

I believe that there is a recursive relationship between the number of physicians and what we define as the boundaries of medicine. Everything that I see now suggests that the boundaries are being expanded because the physicians are available and they are going into whole new fields. The wellness field is part of it, as is plastic surgery for aesthetic purposes. If we have more physicians than necessary, I believe the nature of the system will change.

I think that if a large number of practicing physicians find that they have an insufficient number of patients to satisfy what they believe to be their norm, they will go to their state legislatures and begin to exert pressure on them to help reduce the trend. We pay too little attention to the states, which are, after all, the major payors of medical education in this society. My feeling is that the physicians in active practice will lean against the state legislatures.

I do not believe fundamentally that an American public that is interested in choice will increasingly walk away from choice when it comes to choosing their physicians.

I was dubious about Dr. Ellwood's figures in the early seventies and I am dubious about the figures that have been mentioned here. I do not think we can postulate that all the physicians who do not belong to HMOs are going to do nothing. They are going to do a lot of things and we have no notion how that is going to play out.

DR. RICHARD H. EGDAHL: One group of individuals becoming more and more interested in the quality of medical care are hospital trustees who have the ultimate responsibility for what goes on in hospitals. A few years ago we were approached by a group of hospital trustees from three community hospitals in Massachusetts. They were worried about the figures that show that we have too many surgeons. Many communities have such a surplus of surgeons that the trustees and the hospital management plan to do a lot less surgery than they used to. They also have surplus physicians who do family practice, and it has become apparent that they are doing things they have not been trained to do. This was a great concern to those hospital trustees so they asked us, "Could you help us to devise a manpower model?"

Because hospital medical staffs certify credentials, it has to be the trustees and hospital management looking at this question. I think you will see ever-increasing efforts on the part of hospital trustees to find objective evidence to consider themselves — especially if they are trustees of a community hospital—as a multispecialty group practice. Their doctors are, in effect, practicing fee-for-service medicine in small groups. The trustees are asking for help because they have a quality problem they must be stewards of and there is really no way for them to do these things at the moment.

MR. JACK K. SHELTON: Have the manpower planners taken into consideration the increasing number of licensed nonphysician providers? In many states these providers, who compete with physicians, are getting increased protection to participate in the health care delivery and reimbursement system. These podiatrists, chiropractors, optometrists, nurse practitioners, and others have the ability to generate or reduce demand.

DR. ROBERT G. PETERSDORF: The specialty maldistribution may be even worse than we have been led to believe. You can manipulate the number by looking at the certification process of the American Board of Internal Medicine. The ABIM finds that 70 percent of the people they initially certify sit a subspecialty examination, of whom 50 percent pass. I suggest that the 50 percent who fail are self-declared subspecialists. They never admit publicly that they flunked the examination; in fact, two years later they take it again.

If you look at the other end of it, among the physicians who go into general internal medicine after their residency some go into chief residencies, others go into the service or do other things and then return to do subspecialty fellowships. I think the number who actually come out after three years of training and begin to practice as general internists is probably close to 30 percent, not 39 percent.

MS. MARGARET MAHONEY: I believe that one way change occurs is by word getting out to those who may go into medical specialties. As I understand it, there has been a leveling off of applications to medical school and some medical schools are reducing the number of students they accept. When I go around to campuses I find it interesting to hear the bright young students who might have gone into medicine talking about what other alternatives there are. When you start talking about a surplus publicly and it appears in the newspapers, changes can occur that are really beyond our control. I think we should remember how change occurs.

DR. JOHN A. D. COOPER: The peak in the number of applicants to medical school came in 1974 when there were about 2.8 applicants per physician at that time. Starting in 1974 the number of white male applicants began to drop and it has continued to drop ever since. A little earlier than 1974 the number of women applicants started to rise and continued to rise until this last year and is now plateauing. The women entered the picture and kept our applicant pool from falling as rapidly as it might have. Now, however, with the number of women applicants plateauing and the number of male applicants still decreasing, we have about 32,000 applicants as compared with about 42,000 at the peak. We predict that there will be a further drop in the number of applicants.

Of more concern to us are the more minute details of the states and their applicant pools. In some states medical schools are limited to accepting state residents as students. Some states are already getting into trouble; in Oregon, for example, the applicant pool was not adequate and they did not fill the class. I am concerned about Texas and Arkansas and a few other states as well. We may face the real problem of lacking an adequate number of applicants for medical schools to maintain the class size that they have established.

The applicants themselves may play an important role in deciding how many physicians we educate and train. Young people are hearing that there are too many physicians, that they are not going to make as much money, and that they are in the wrong specialties and practicing in the wrong places. After they hear enough of this they may well decide to go into business or some other area.

DR. DAVID SATCHER: Those of us who are involved in and concerned with education of minorities, especially blacks, in medicine are especially concerned with the projection of oversupply and the reaction to it. There are two reasons for our concern: one, there is still a significant underrepresentation of minorities in medicine, especially blacks, who comprise significantly less than 3 percent; two, the pressure that is being brought to bear to reduce the enrollment of students in medical schools is probably felt disproportionately by minorities. If you take just the increase in tuition and decrease in capitation, these forces have impacted upon blacks in medicine more severely than upon others. Therefore, we are especially concerned with the reaction to the projected surplus.

The fact of the matter is that today the pressures to decrease enrollment have significantly impacted on blacks. At Meharry in 1978, significantly more than 50 percent of the students had National Health Service Corps scholarships. Without question, these scholarships meant far more to black students as a way of paying their way through medical school than they did to other students. Seventy-five percent of Meharry graduates have chosen to practice in underserved inner-city and rural communities, and the fact that their commitment to the National Health Service Corps in return for their scholarships was to go to those communities was a natural. Because it was really especially attractive to black students, the discontinuation of the National Health Service Corps has had a major impact upon black students in medical school. I think those things need to be kept in mind if, in fact, we are concerned with equal opportunity of access to medical education in this country.

At Meharry the enrollment of women has approached 50 percent for quite a while, and it is now 44 percent in the residency program. That is not surprising when we consider the fact that when Daniel Patrick Moynihan did his study back in the early sixties, he pointed out that almost 65 percent of the blacks in colleges at that time were women. There are a lot of cultural factors related to that in terms of the black community and the role of women as compared with men.

MR. WILLIS GOLDBECK: It seems to me that medical education is caught up in a much larger problem than numbers. That problem is what I would posit as a gap between the structure and results of professional education in general in the United States on the one hand and the society in which those professionals are going to have to work for, presumably, a very long period of time on the other. We see many of the same problems in business schools and law schools: attempting to turn out people who have even a reasonably close understanding of what business or law is going to be twenty years from now. This is not something that is strictly a medical education issue.

Look at the fact that the society we are dealing with is one in which only one-tenth of the households have a man at work and a woman at home with a child. This problem goes a long way beyond medical school, and almost none of our educational institutions or work institutions have any understanding of what to do about it.

Cultural problems extend way beyond those you have heard until now. The major growth of the population in the United States is Hispanic and Asian and Islamic; it is nonoccidental in its cultural heritage. Its definitions of death are different. Its definitions of the role of man in society are different. It has very different basic parameters for the kinds of things that are important to people. What are the professional schools doing about the fact that there will be a significant demand from people in their forties and fifties to go to professional schools? At that point they will have finished one or two careers and are not going to die on cue at sixty-five but are going to be living until eighty-five, with twenty more years to contribute to society. The attraction of a high-quality, professional life-style and the contributions a professional person can make are going to be just as attractive to people in their forties and fifties as it is today to people in their twenties when the motivations and understandings of what those careers might lead to are very different.

I would like to suggest that what we are discussing is part of a much larger setting of societal and other related issues than we can resolve just by trying to balance out the numbers on a chart.

DR. ROBERT H. MOSER: I want to ask Dr. Satcher if the batting average for retention of black physicians by National Health Service Corps has been good.

DR. DAVID SATCHER: I do not know if the figure is still 75 percent. I doubt that we had the same kind of dropout of blacks from underserved communities as there was of whites. There are reasons for that. Most of our students come from those communities in the first place, so going back to them is not quite the same as asking people to go to communities that are foreign to them. It is more natural for them to go to the inner cities and the rural areas.

MR. PAUL G. ROGERS: It was never the intent of that legislation for physicians to go into underserved areas and stay forever. We did expect them to stay two, three, or four years and then to be replaced by others coming in. We never anticipated that they would fill the gaps of the underserved areas other than by replacement. That was the intent of the legislation.

DR. ALVIN R. TARLOV: I would like Professor Enthoven to respond to the question about HMOs skimming the healthier population. Does the analysis of the HMO data need to take into account the fact that the enrollees in HMOs are healthier by and large than the individuals in the first compartment?

PROFESSOR ALAIN C. ENTHOVEN: Yes, with respect to both physicians and hospital beds. You do have to consider age-specific doctor/office visit rates and bed utilization rates. It would probably be appropriate for Dr. Ellwood to make some adjustments for that in his figures.

DR. PAUL M. ELLWOOD, JR.: We have found, surprisingly, that as people grow old in HMOs, their hospital utilization rates and visit rates drop.

DR. ALVIN R. TARLOV: I wonder whether Dr. Nesbitt feels that the calculations need to take into account the growth in nonphysician health care providers that began in the seventies.

DR TOM E. NESBITT: One of the five panels that studied the GMENAC activities was devoted to the nonphysician health care providers. It was our conclusion that the number of these health care providers was not likely to increase significantly. We concluded that they would play a diminishing role except for optometrists, and they were a subject we did not have the time or resources to explore as much as we would have liked. The role of the nurse practitioner and particularly the nurse midwife was explored in some depth. The nurse midwives came back to us in the course of our final considerations when they found that there was no way that they could develop their schools to create enough nurse practitioners to meet the obstetrical care needs that we had already assigned to them.

It is my feeling that GMENAC adequately pursued and studied the areas of nonphysician health care providers.

DR. ALVIN R. TARLOV: I would hope that we might be willing to just accept the fact that the supply of physicians is growing at a certain rate relative to the population and concentrate instead on the meaning of that growth. What effect should it have on curriculum and the way we select individuals for medical school? What effect is it going to have on the quality of practice?

What does it mean when we have 600,000 patients with acute myocardial infarctions each year, 300,000 of whom die before they get to a hospital? What does it mean when 170,000 of the remaining

300,000 are having coronary artery surgery at an annual expenditure of $4 billion? What does it mean in terms of the growth of the physician supply, particularly of cardiologists? What does it mean when the density of cardiologists in the first compartment is twelve times greater than in the third compartment? What effect will that fact have on the incidence of coronary artery bypass surgery?

I think there are a lot of social issues involved in the physician surplus. The response to the growing supply of physicians has been surprisingly constructive in some segments. The medical schools are beginning to respond to it in a way that they think is appropriate. On the other hand, the teaching hospitals have not responded appropriately in the distribution of their training physicians. It would be good to examine why they have not. What are the forces that prevent the teaching hospitals from taking a more aggressive stand in examining the issues and trying to respond to them?

We ought not to focus on deciding whether or not there is a surplus. Rather we should just understand that the growth rate is rather steep, that this in itself will have some effects, and that other changes are happening in terms of technology, in terms of life-style aspirations, and in terms of placing some limit on the expenditures that we are willing to make for health care. What would be constructive responses to these issues?

2

The University's Role in Establishing Priorities for Medical Education: A Societal Perspective

WILLIAM H. DANFORTH, M.D.

We in the United States are quite fond of allocating responsibility and even more fond of allocating blame. If I were an investigative reporter trying to fix blame for the shortcomings I saw in American medicine, I wonder where I would fix it? I would ask myself such questions as: What institutions educate most of the medical students and many premedical students? What institutions set the standards that have such an effect on all premedical curricula and on the behavior of premedical students? What is the institutional affiliation of those who oversee residency programs and have such a major influence on the standards of specialty boards? Where is the most biomedical research done? Where is most thought given to reorganizational improvement?

The facts are, first, that the universities are a directly dominant influence on the lives of young people heading for medical practice from about age eighteen to thirty-one and, second, in the last years of that period the teaching hospitals set the standards and styles for newly minted physicians. No other professional school is involved in this way. When a business student receives the MBA, he or she moves to a business organization, hopefully continuing to learn but outside the domain of the university; a new law graduate may clerk for a judge or may go directly into practice; but a budding young surgeon receives an M.D. degree and he or she will likely be found reporting to the head of the university's department of surgery, who also serves as chief of the hospital surgical services. Even after leaving the residency the young physician may continue an affiliation with the university and, if not, will certainly have his or her practice affected by the research and the ideas coming out of medical school.

Another difference in medical education is that nowhere else in the university is there talk of limits. We would be glad to train all the historians who wanted training at Washington University. We are happy to train lawyers in large numbers. We are concerned about quality, of course, but that is just one institution's concern. A group in St. Louis is starting a new law school. No thought has been given to the need for more lawyers; rather this new school is fulfilling a demand for places for people who want to have legal training. That goes on in most of our universities. Yet we deal with medical education in a very different way.

Most of us have a sense of responsibility for our students. We want to maximize their options, not to limit them. As Americans we are prone to expect too much from our educational institutions. I am glad that I work for an institution from which much is expected and I think it is incumbent on us to look on that expectation as an opportunity and do what we can to be helpful.

What should society be asking of universities? Realistically we know that our institutions cannot solve all the problems of medical care. What should we, in turn, want the larger society to ask of us? I think we have two major charges: one is to do our best to educate the physicians for the future, and the second is to provide the intellectual and scientific leadership that will allow our children and grandchildren to fare better than we.

Will American universities and their schools of medicine be responsive to the needs, aspirations, and ethical standards of society in educating future physicians? The answer, I believe, is generally yes. American medical schools have in the past responded to societal expectations by changing, and changing very drastically. The major changes have usually occurred after there is consensus on what the change ought to be; they have occurred as a result of cooperation between medical schools and other agencies of society, for example, medical education following the Flexner report, the growth of biomedical research after World War II and its incorporation in the curriculum, the expansion of medical school class size, and so on. There is responsiveness. Sometimes the ideas for things we want to have happen come out of the universities and then come back to us through either legislation or outside funding.

The problem in dealing with numbers is that with more than one hundred medical schools, it is hard to respond coherently unless there is a widespread consensus. Outside forces can very much affect individual institutions and, if those forces get very large, they can influence a number of us. Washington University has just cut back on the enrollment in the School of Dental

Medicine, not because there are too many dentists but because we have too few applicants. It is very difficult for a young dentist from Missouri to get a loan from a bank to start up an independent practice. The banks do not feel the individual can pay off the loan without a lot of luck and/or outside income.

I do not believe that voluntary restraint on the part of institutions that train medical students will work. There is too much hubris in individual departments which feel they are too great to cut back and too much advantage in being the last to cut back to make that a very workable solution.

Individual institutions, on the other hand, can address perceived shortcomings in the whole spectrum of American medical education. Several shortcomings have been identified recently by thoughtful individuals and by groups: there is continuing erosion of the general education of physicians; the admissions requirements are having a baleful and malign effect on undergraduate education; young physicians should have better writing skills and more understanding of medical history and economics, as well as better training in management, statistics, and information sciences; medical education is poorly organized and the curriculum overly dense; students are required to memorize too many facts in medical schools; students are not encouraged to develop analytic and synthetic skills or to study independently; greater effort should be made to pass on appropriate values and attitudes for physicians and to evaluate personal characteristics of medical students or potential medical students; greater and more prolonged contact is needed between individual students and faculty members so as to provide more effective mentors or models; and new organizational structures are needed in order to oversee teaching, with separate budgets for these organizational structures.

These criticisms are not trivial; many of them are aimed at making fundamental changes in what we do. Nor are these criticisms hostile; they are made by our friends.

I have thought about ways that we might proceed at our institution, and one I intend to explore is the idea of setting up a group charged with thinking hard about medical education from the standpoint of the individual being educated. I would envision such a group including faculty from arts and sciences, medicine, and engineering and containing persons knowledgeable in educational methods and learning theory. Such a group would need to be familiar with the recent evaluations of medical education and the many innovative practices throughout the nation. The difficult question of how to provide a basic core of knowledge to all physicians while also providing more varied careers that so many see in the future is not going to be easy to answer. We need room for those with special interests in philosophy, politics, biochemistry, management, statistics, engineering, economics, and so on.

I make this rather modest suggestion with the assumption that it is not time for a new Flexner report to change radically what we should be doing in schools of medicine. It is a time for thinking, for experimentation, for trial and error, and for evaluation. It is doubtful even that we want one model for medical education; we probably want more diversity in the future. I think this era calls for courage for different institutions to try new forms that engender criticism or skepticism. It also requires humility to recognize that one cannot be certain of the best form of medical education and that one can learn from others.

If we are to experiment and to encourage experimentation, we need to be very flexible in our selection procedures so as to allow for experimentation. We must be able to evaluate our individual processes and procedures and the results of our educational process better than we do. We need to collect data and to evaluate progress and outcomes; we also need to tackle difficult questions about the appropriateness of our selection procedures, the standards of grading, and the encouragement of appropriate behavior.

The second major change is to provide intellectual and scientific leadership that will allow our grandchildren to do better than we do. I think all of us are convinced of the importance of medical and biomedical science although we all have problems in doing it well, given cost and subsidization changes.

There is clearly more need for research into the human side of the delivery of health care—for example, the effectiveness of physicians; the personal characteristics that lead to effectiveness; models of practice and how they affect outcomes, management, and costs; management of health care resources; the effect of economic incentives on medical practice; and improved methods for aiding physicians by computer networks and for determining how these aids can be tied into continuing education. If our institutions would do more research in these areas it would not only be helpful in understanding some of the problems we are talking about today, but it would also give us a better understanding of what medical education should lead to. It would give us a different kind of person serving on our curriculum committees and make medical education much better.

Finally, I think a study of our educational processes is in order. What I am suggesting is not something new but a greatly enlarged effort and, I hope, an enlarged partnership between our universities and some funding agencies in this endeavor.

Managing Quality and Quantity in Residency Training Programs

JOHN S. GRAETTINGER, M.D.

I would like to show you a few selected items out of the report of the 1985 residency matching program and suggest three things: one, we have an excess number of PGY-1 positions; two, there is a lack of congruence among the specialties perceived to be in short supply, in excess supply, and the aspirations of students; three, some programs are only slightly used for the graduate medical education of U.S. medical school students.

In the 1985 match there were 18,500 positions, an increase of only about one hundred, mainly in internal medicine. U.S. seniors have increased only about 1 percent a year since 1980 and there will be about 16,300 this year. There is, then, a 1.14 ratio of positions to students, that is, an excess of positions.

Besides U.S. seniors who seek PGY-1 positions, there are others who seek entry. These include a modest number of Canadians: 200. They also include previous years' graduates of our own schools; over the last three years, the number of previous years' graduates recycling and seeking a position in competition with seniors has gone up about fourfold. Osteopaths have been included at a rate of about 200 a year until two years ago, when the output of new osteopathic schools reached the stage where their internship positions did not keep pace, and now 600 osteopathic graduates seek allopathic residencies. There are also about 400 fifth-pathway students. Finally, included in the U.S. citizens are those who have enrolled in the unaccredited proprietary schools ringing the Caribbean Sea. In 1981 there were 700; in 1982 there were twice as many; in 1983, 2,000; and in 1984, 3,000. This year, their numbers decreased by 300.

Last, there is the greatest single number outside the U.S. seniors, namely non-U.S. citizen foreign medical school graduates. In 1976, when total applicants first reached 20,000, there were 6,000 alien graduates. Then came the Visa Qualifying Examination and a decrement in total and then an astonishing rise. In July 1984 the Foreign Medical Graduate Examination in the Medical Sciences (FMGEMS) was instituted and, whether or not causally, the number of alien graduates was down by 200 this year. All in all, we had 28,000 applicants for some 18,500 positions.

What happens to this vast group? Figure 9 shows the ratio of positions to applicants and the number of unmatched applicants. This year the percentage of our unmatched U.S. senior students decreased from 7.8 to 7.4. Fifth-pathway students, who have had a supervised clinical year, had 18.8 percent unmatched this year. After U.S. seniors, they and Canadians are the most preferred applicants by program directors.

The unmatched USFMG went to 60 percent this year. They clearly have suffered with the drop in the position/applicant ratio. The unmatched rate of alien FMGs is inversely related to the position/applicant ratio: 78.4 percent went unmatched this year, up from last year.

The second point I want to discuss is the matter of congruence of aspirations of our students and kinds of positions. Overall, 13 percent of U.S. students did not get their specialty of first choice:

Figure 9. Ratio of Physicians to Applicants and the Number of Unmatched Applicants.

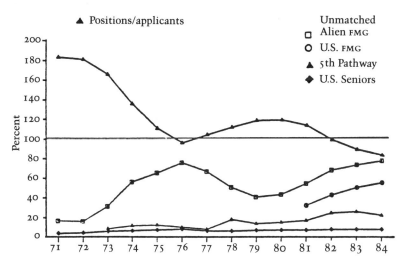

7.2 percent who listed family practice as their first choice did not get it; 25 percent of those who listed obstetrics and gynecology first did not get it; in general surgery, 14 percent; in the surgical specialties, 41 percent; in anesthesiology, 26 percent; in emergency medicine, nearly 40 percent; and in radiology, one-third. In other words, although the number of positions is adequate, it is perfectly obvious that student aspirations are not being met by the positions offered. I do not say they should be but that they are not being.

Finally, I would like to point out something about the 3,000 empty positions. Three-quarters of the 18,500 positions were filled by LCME graduates and another 11 percent by others, but there were 2,262 empty positions or 12 percent of the total offered. Figure 10 divides all the positions available into three categories, based on their being filled by U.S. senior students. In group A were 66 percent of the programs and positions, which filled 75 to 100 percent of their positions with U.S. seniors. The mean filling of these programs by LCME graduates was 97 percent, only 2 percent non-LCME graduates, and 1 percent of the positions remained empty. These programs in group A contained 84 percent of the

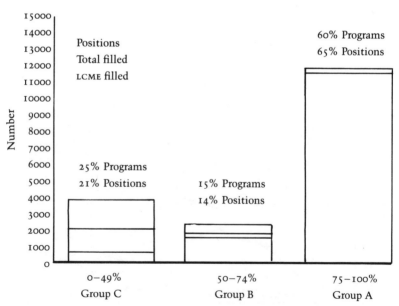

Figure 10. Positions Available, by Category, Filled by U.S. Senior Students.

LCME graduates who matched, only 12 percent of non-LCME graduates, and only 6 percent of the total empty positions.

In group C there were some 3,900 positions in one-fifth of the programs that filled less than 50 percent of their positions with U.S. seniors. The mean filling of these programs by LCME graduates was only 20 percent, with another 40 percent filled by others, but 40 percent of their positions were empty. In other words, these programs attracted only 6 percent of LCME graduates, three-quarters of the non-LCME, and contained three-quarters of the empty positions.

On the basis of the AAMC and NRMP follow-up studies, we can confidently predict that the thousand unmatched graduates will go into group A, group B, and a few group C positions. But there will be some 1,500 positions unfilled by LCME graduates, which I submit serve as a vacuum into which other graduates will flow.

In sum, if we have about 16,000 graduates and about 20,000 positions, we have some 4,000 positions that are not being used by our graduates and that serve as the vacuum into which other graduates flow. It is interesting that in 1968 Dr. Tarlov said it would be 4,100.

The Impact of State Licensing Boards on the Distribution and Quality of Physicians

BRYANT L. GALUSHA, M.D.

Medical licensing boards are not directly involved in physician supply and distribution; however, they are involved with quality issues which indirectly affect supply and distribution. Therefore, I will discuss licensing boards' impact on quality and point out their coincidental impact on the distribution and supply of physicians.

In the broadest terms, state medical boards are charged by state statute with the responsibility of regulating the practice of medicine and surgery. In general, state medical boards have two major areas of responsibility: that of licensure and that of disciplinary action. In the area of licensure, boards have the power to award, deny, suspend, or revoke a license. In exercising any of these options, boards again are concerned with quality.

The ever-present question in the minds of board members interviewing an applicant for licensure or confronting a physician whose license is in jeopardy is, Can this physician practice medicine with reasonable skill and safety?

There are presently four general prerequisites required by boards for the granting of a license to practice medicine. The candidate for licensure must possess acceptable personal attributes, have successfully completed the curriculum of a medical school approved by the board, have obtained a passing grade on a medical licensing examination, and demonstrate clinical competency as evidenced by satisfactory completion of one or more years of approved graduate medical education.

The graduate medical education requirement, which is clearly a quality assurance requirement, possibly could be interpreted as a manpower control factor, especially today. Obviously, if a graduate of a school of medicine cannot obtain a residency position in an approved graduate medical education program, he or she cannot be licensed. This clearly affects foreign medical graduates. As Dr. Graettinger pointed out, there are not enough positions to satisfy the demands of the total pool of GME applicants made up of U.S. graduates, USFMGS, and foreign national FMGS. Therefore, the graduate medical education requirement for licensure may well be viewed by many as a manpower control factor and, in fact, as an exercise in discrimination.

Presently only three state medical licensing boards require more than one year of graduate medical education for graduates of LCME-accredited medical schools. However, an increasing number of states are requiring three years of graduate medical education for foreign medical graduates. The increased graduate medical education requirement for the foreign medical graduate is a quality assurance measure put in place partly to compensate for the lack of a clear insight into the quality of the undergraduate medical education of many foreign medical schools. The extended graduate medical education requirement provides licensing boards with more opportunity to evaluate the medical knowledge and performance of the foreign medical graduate applicant. I believe one can safely say that the licensing boards' requirement for a prescribed period of graduate medical education does have an influence on the quality of practicing physicians.

Medical licensing boards affect the quality of physicians by requiring the passage of one of two reliable and valid tests of medical knowledge: the Federation Licensing Examination, the so-called FLEX examination, or the National Board of Medical Examiners' examination sequence. The advent in 1968 of the Federation Licensing Examination made a most significant change in the licensing process in this country. State boards, through their federation, had available for use as their state examination a uniform, reliable, valid, and high-quality test instrument. Many state licensing examinations prior to 1968 were, at best, marginal test instruments; a number of states through the years did not have a single failure. The FLEX program was developed because state licensing boards recognized, for quality assurance reasons, the need for a valid and reliable licensure examination. By states insisting on reliable and valid examinations for licensure, they are having a significant effect on the overall quality of practicing physicians.

It is also worthy of mention that acceptance of the FLEX examination program by all states and other licensing jurisdictions as their own examination allowed for a rational basis for reciprocity and licensure by endorsement between states. This has favorably affected distribution by providing greater freedom of interstate movement by physicians.

The process of licensure involves significant credentialing responsibilities for licensing boards. These credentialing responsibilities also affect physician quality. Usually, when dealing with graduates of LCME-accredited medical schools, the evaluation of personal attributes and undergraduate medical education borders on purposeless motion and is routine to the point of boredom. Unfortunately, such a situation can lead to laxity and to the award of a license to an unfit individual.

The granting of a license is a relatively effortless procedure when compared with the time, expense, and frustration of trying to retrieve or revoke one. I speak from experience of twelve years on the North Carolina Board of Medical Examiners when I say that proper credentialing procedures carried out by medical licensing boards are necessary quality assurance measures and must be done thoroughly for all applicants.

The major credentialing problems presently confronting licensing boards involve graduates of many of the new foreign medical schools, especially those targeted toward the training of U.S. citizens. Boards find it difficult to obtain reliable information from these schools on which to make sound licensure decisions. Legitimate diplomas cannot be totally relied upon to guarantee the adequacy of undergraduate medical education, nor can reference letters from faculty members, regardless of how glowing they are, be interpreted as adequate testimony to an applicant's personal attributes. This unenviable position in which licensing boards now find themselves has been further aggravated by the present despicable problem of fraudulent medical education credentials. The federation, in response to requests of the state medical licensing boards, recently appointed an ad hoc committee to study this problem. This committee was charged with the responsibility of developing a proposal for identifying such credentials, protecting against their successful use, exposing their use, and cooperating with state and federal law enforcement agencies in taking appropriate legal action against the imposters. As a result of this task force's work and its recommendations and the efforts of individual licensing boards, boards are now instituting elaborate credential checking for all graduates, especially those of the foreign medical schools. Several boards have declared a moratorium on consideration of applicants from certain schools. Many boards have refused applicants the privilege of taking the licensing examination because the quality of their undergraduate medical education could not be documented. In fact, the North Carolina Board of Medical Examiners was involved in a prolonged legal action for denying the graduates of St. George's Medical School the privilege of sitting for the North Carolina examination. These actions and others by licensing boards can be cited as having an impact on the quality of the practicing physicians.

Some states must now or in the near future consider for license examination the graduates of many schools of unknown quality. Facing this possibility, the member boards of the federation have mandated that the federation establish a commission charged with the collection and validation of data to help states make judgments on the educational programs of specified foreign medical schools. The federation is responding to this mandate and has received the legal authority to serve as a fact-finding body for all fifty-four medical licensing jurisdictions of this country and its territories. The information that the federation's commission will gather and validate will be passed on to the individual licensing boards for their own evaluation in approving or disapproving those medical education programs for licensure purposes. This too will have an impact on the quality of practicing physicians, one that all of us hope will be favorable.

There are several other procedures by which licensing boards affect the quality of physicians. The majority of boards require all applicants for licensure to have a personal interview with either the board as a whole, a board member, or the executive secretary of the board. The personal interview is considered by most boards to be a valuable screening procedure; occasionally it can result in the outright denial of a license or the withholding of a license pending further documentation of credentials, cognitive knowledge, competence, and/or acceptable character.

There is an increasing trend toward more detailed evaluation of the physician seeking a license via the endorsement/reciprocity route. In addition to a personal interview, many state licensing boards have adopted formal examination procedures. For example, Texas requires that the applicant who has not taken a licensing examination during the past three years pass the clinical competency portion of the FLEX examination. Oregon requires an oral examination for all physicians who have been out of residency training for more than five years and are not certified by a specialty board.

Alabama, in addition to using the FLEX, requires a formal oral examination for all foreign medical graduates unless they have been certified or recertified by an ABMS-approved specialty board within the past ten years. Alabama also requires an oral exam for all U.S. graduates who have not passed either the National Board sequence or the FLEX within a ten-year period. North Carolina and many other states have used the spontaneous oral examination as a screen to obtain more formal documentation of cognitive knowledge or competence.

The granting of a medical license is only the beginning of the medical board's responsibilities. Equally important is the board's obligation to protect the public from licensed physicians who are not practicing medicine with reasonable skill and safety. The disciplinary duties of medical boards are by and large inordinately time consuming, frustrating, and distressing for board members; however, on occasion, they can be professionally rewarding.

In dealing with deviant physicians, most of the board's work is done under a cloak of confidentiality, using an informal hearing where a physician is invited to appear before the board to explain the findings of a board's investigative staff in response to a specific allegation against the physician. This can vary from a minor and easily correctable aberration in prescribing habits to major infractions such as gross misconduct or incompetence. The former can be handled frequently by simply bringing to the attention of the physician the potential seriousness of his or her deviant behavior coupled with identification of the specific remedial action the board expects, such as a prescription-monitoring program. The latter may well result in a cease and desist order by the board with the drawing up of formal charges for a public hearing before the board, the most serious consequence being revocation of the charged physician's license.

Occasionally the informal disciplinary proceedings of the board can be most satisfying and rewarding. Probably all seasoned members of licensing boards have had the exhilarating experience of helping several basically good physicians correct some bad professional and/or personal habits that could have resulted ultimately in severe professional sanctions and possibly significant public harm if they had gone undetected. I could cite examples of physicians, including residents, young practicing physicians, academicians of all ranks, and elderly physicians who have served their communities with distinction for many years, who were saved from professional and personal embarrassment by a board's identifying and assisting them in correcting a long list of deviances that could have led to catastrophic results.

For every physician disciplinary encounter with a board that results in formal charges, there are at least fifteen to twenty informal hearings. Clearly, the disciplinary activities of medical boards affect physician quality, not only in each board's respective state but nationwide.

The federation has a computerized disciplinary data bank that collects and stores all disciplinary actions taken against physicians resulting from formal charges. This information is reviewed, categorized, and distributed monthly to all U.S. and territorial licensing authorities, all of which are members of the federation, to the American Medical Association for use in their physician master file data base, to the American Osteopathic Association, to the Department of Health and Human Services Office of Financial Integrity, and to many other appropriate agencies and institutions. The disciplinary data bank's effectiveness is now being demonstrated almost daily. It is becoming increasingly difficult for physicians who have been disciplined in one state to move to another undetected. It is difficult for disciplined physicians to seek haven in the armed forces or for a physician dismissed from the armed forces because of incompetence or a character defect to enter civilian practice undetected. This collective cooperation of medical licensing boards, through their federation, is also having a significant effect on the quality of licensed physicians.

Individuals who voluntarily serve as members of state licensing and disciplinary boards, be they physicians or be they laymen, make a significant personal sacrifice to serve the public good. They are frequently faulted when the fault is often not theirs but rather the result of insufficient financial support to fulfill their public responsibilities and of restrictions imposed by inadequate state medical practice acts. Working with its member licensing boards, the federation is making a concerted effort to encourage sufficient funding for licensing and disciplinary boards and to provide guidelines for modern state medical practice acts, which, in turn, can be expected to positively affect the practice of medicine throughout the nation.

The Experience in Great Britain
JOHN LISTER, M.D.

The rather uniform pattern of health care provided by the National Health Service (NHS) in Great Britain presents an enormous contrast to the heterogeneous system in this country. Our present government is encouraging the private sector, but it remains small, caring for somewhere between 5 and 7 percent of the population. For 90 percent of the population the NHS remains the way in which they get access to health care. The NHS provides access to the health care system for anyone requiring treatment, regardless of their means; it provides minimal acceptable standards and often something very much better than that.

I recently attended a conference at the Royal College of Physicians on priorities in medicine. Two of the major topics were finance and the adequacy of care. The message was that we in Britain must recognize that we are a relatively poor country, unlikely to be able to spend more than the present 6 percent of our GDP for the NHS. We must therefore go in pursuit of obtaining value for money. Thus the emphasis in Great Britain at the present time is on management efficiency and the identification of priorities.

Forecasting medical manpower needs is notoriously difficult, and there is obviously no single answer to the question of how many doctors we need. The ratio of doctors to population is certainly not a reliable indicator of need since the normally accepted indicators of health show no definite correlation with the number of doctors in practice. Nevertheless, the doctor/population quotient has shown a steady rise in all developed countries. The rate of increase in this quotient in Great Britain since the beginning of the century has been 1.25 percent per annum.

The answer to the question of how many doctors we need

depends on many factors: the future role of physicians; the increasing number of women doctors who may wish to work part-time; the changing patterns of disease; the life-styles of doctors; the impact of medical and scientific advances; changing demography; and the increasing longevity of the population. But in our country, and probably in all countries in the end, the ultimate determining factor may be the availability of resources. So the question is, How many doctors can we afford?

Most of the factors mentioned apply equally to any developed country, but in Britain there are a number of special factors.

General Background

Figure 11 shows how the doctor/population quotient has gone steadily up in Britain. In the year 2000, we will need something over 100,000 doctors in Great Britain. We have in England, Wales, Scotland, and Northern Ireland a total population of 54.4 million, one-fifth of the size of the population of the United States. Thus, if you multiply anything I say by five you will achieve some degree of comparability between our two countries.

The British problems we have to consider are, first, the fact that the federal state, in the form of the National Health Service, is the monopoly employer. There are only about 10,000 doctors who are not associated with practice in the NHS. Second, the number of doctors employed is constrained by cash limits and this is a very controlled financial situation now. There is a global budget determined by the Department of the Treasury, given to the Department of Health, and parceled out to the regions, which parcel the money out to districts, of which there are about 200. These authorities are all constrained by cash limits. They have to spend their money in the light of competing claims on priorities.

Third, the rigid career structure for the profession makes things extremely difficult. It is also complicated by fairly rigid training programs. Fourth, in our country, too, we have the FMG problem to which Dr. Asper referred.

In England, the Health Departments are the departments that determine the size of our medical school intake. The Department of Education and Science and the University Grants Committee fund undergraduate medical education and academic postgraduate medical education. The General Medical Council maintains a register of duly qualified practitioners. It was established to enable people to distinguish the qualified from the unqualified practi-

tioner. It is our disciplinary body; it regulates the medical profession. It has the duty of coordinating all aspects of medical
education, including postgraduate and continuing education. The
Royal Colleges and Faculties are the bodies that traditionally have
maintained standards through Higher Training Committees, which
determine the training programs for specialists. We also have
Manpower Committees, central and regional, which determine the
distribution of doctors in the health service. One of our major

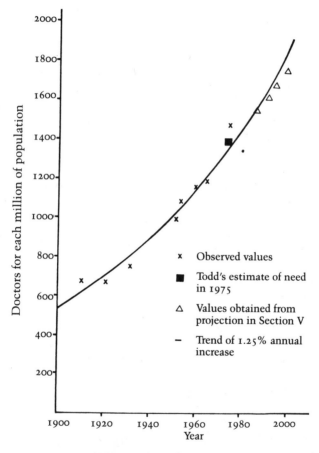

Figure 11. Doctor/Population Quotient in Great Britain.

Source: Reprinted with permission of the Controller of Her Britannic
Majesty's Stationery Office. Department of Health and Social Security,
Medical Manpower—the Next Twenty Years (London: Her Majesty's
Stationery Office, 1982).

problems is balancing the training requirements and the service needs.

Structure of Our Profession

Career structure in Great Britain is somewhat different from that in the United States (Figure 12). The medical graduate in Great Britain must do a one-year internship (six months in general medical subjects, and six months in general surgical subjects) before he becomes fully registered. He is still the responsibility of the medical school for that year after graduation. He then makes his decision whether to become a general practice vocational trainee or a general professional trainee.

At the moment, many decide to go into general practice and do primary care. A unique feature of Britain's NHS is that all of us get access to the health care system through our general practitioner. Today, nearly 50 percent of young graduates will decide to go into general practice and so they seek a rotational program as a vocational trainee. That is a three-year program at the end of which they can seek a place in general practice.

On the other side is the man who wants to become a hospital specialist. He does three years in general professional posts, looking for one post after another because there are not many packages. At the end of that time he will seek a higher professional training post as a senior registrar and that is basically a four-year training

Figure 12. Career Structure

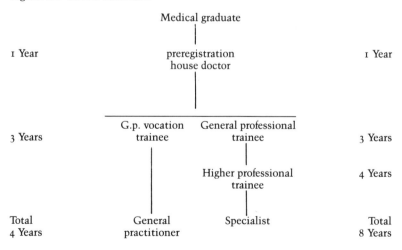

Figure 13. Hospital Staff: England and Wales. *Source: Health Trends 1984*, vol. 16. Figures as of September 1983.

Senior hospital staff Consultants (tenured)	13,631
Senior registrars	3,235 (4-year program)
Registrars	6,183 (3-year program)
SHOS	10,250 (2-year program)

program. At the end of that time he is eligible to seek a specialist or consultant post.

In Britain, there are 28,000 principals in general practice. If you divide them into the 54 million population, there are just about 2,000 patients per general practitioner. The College of General Practitioners would like to get it down to 1,750 per doctor but this is a long way from the HMO figure of 1.1 doctor per thousand.

Figure 13 shows something of the situation with the hospital staff. The only tenured hospital staff, apart from the academic staff who have honorary contracts in the health service, are the senior hospital staff, and we have less than 14,000 of them. Senior registrars, the chief residents, number 3,235, the registrars number 6,183, and the senior house officers number 10,250. If a consultant holds office for twenty-eight years and the senior registrar for four years, then there should be seven consultants to one senior registrar. Unfortunately, that is not the way it is. In the future there will be room for a very small number of tenured people.

Figure 14 shows the FMG problem. There are not many FMGs in the preregistration year (house officers). We do not encourage them to come to Great Britain until they are eligible to get on the medical register in some way or other. At least 50 percent of the senior house officers are FMGs and over 50 percent of the registrars. There is a smaller number of them among the senior registrars. Not very many get permanently absorbed into tenured posts.

We have a situation, then, where half of the people in training posts are FMGs. We do not know quite how many go home, but it may be 80 percent eventually. Many of them are in the less-desirable posts.

The numbers of consultants and senior registrars in some of the popular specialties in Britain are quite different from the situation in the United States. We only have 1,122 general internists, 942 general surgeons, 557 pediatricians, 167 urologists, and 92 neurosurgeons, but they do different work from what is done in this country. If you multiply these numbers by five you will see how they compare with the United States.

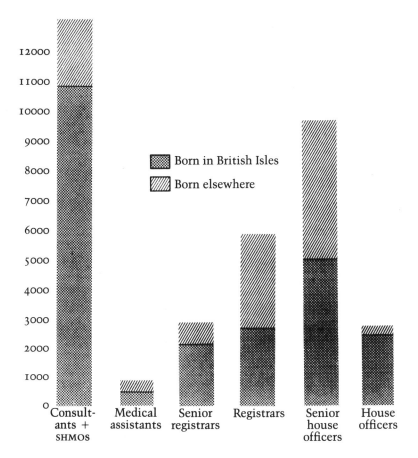

Figure 14. Numbers of Doctors in Each Grade by Place of Birth: England and Wales. *Source*: House of Commons Report, *Medical Education* (London: Her Majesty's Stationery Office, 1982). Figures as of September 1980. Reprinted with permission of the Controller of Her Britannic Majesty's Stationery Office.

Training Programs and Career Prospects

The general practitioners have done a good deal to improve training for their practice of primary medicine, but I think it was unfortunate to get legislation passed so that in order to become a principal in general practice in Great Britain, you must have done certain trainings. It is the only branch of the profession where the actual training program is on the statute books.

Training for a general practice is a three-year program after the preregistration year, followed by two years in rotating posts in appropriate departments, and then one year as a trainee in an approved practice with an approved trainer. One of the problems is that you have to make the decision to go into this form of practice fairly early; if you fail to get up the ladder of whatever specialty you chose, it is increasingly difficult to double back, because you may not have done many of the required training slots.

Persons aspiring to become hospital consultants go through the years of medical school, preclinical study, clinical study, the preregistration year, general professional training, and higher professional training for a total of fourteen years. At the age of thirty-two they should have completed their higher professional training and got accreditation in the specialty of their choice. As it stands in many specialties, people do not get appointed to their consultant posts until the age of about thirty-eight.

In Britain the Royal Colleges are the standard-setting bodies. They determine the training programs for all the specialties. The Royal College of Physicians of London and Edinburgh and Glasgow has a committee called the Joint Committee on Higher Medical Training, and there are twenty specialty advisory committees which draw up the training programs that senior registrars have to follow before they can get accredited. No hospital is allowed to appoint a senior registrar to a post unless it has had its training program approved so that the individual will be eligible for accreditation at the end. The Colleges also conduct entry examinations into higher training, membership of the College of Physicians, fellowship of the College of Surgeons, and membership of the College of Obstetrics and Gynecology and of Psychiatry.

Each region has a Senior Registrar Training Committee, which looks after the senior registrars in posts throughout the region. However, the creation of a post depends on two other factors: educational clearance by one of the higher training committees and manpower clearance by the Central or Regional Manpower

Committee. The number of senior registrars is strictly controlled and is supposed to be in balance with the number of consultant vacancies.

How Many Doctors?

We come down again to the question of how many doctors. We have expended great efforts in England to determine how many we need. There was the 1944 Goodenough Committee which esti- mated that the annual entry of 2,500 students would lead to 50,000 doctors by 1953 but, in fact, by the late forties, the annual intake was only 2,000. Then we had the very famous Willink Committee in 1957 which recommended a major cut to 1,760 students annually. The thing we always have to remember is that there is a five or six year latent period after changing the number before the effect comes along. Fortunately, before the effect came along it was recognized that the Willink Committee had made a mistake by not realizing that there would be a great deal of medical emigra- tion at that time. Nor had it realized that there was going to be a miscalculation on population numbers, and a miscalculation on the fact that the health service was in an expansive mood so that there were to be an increased number of career opportunities.

In 1961 the University Grants Committee and the Department of Health recommended an increase in the medical school intake. The 1965 Todd Commission recommended a further increase in intake. In 1978 there was a very good report by the Department of Health which recommended increasing the intake figure to 4,080 by 1983–84; if you multiply that by five, you see that is quite a large number of intake even relative to that of the United States. In 1980 another report reaffirmed the 4,080. The Short Report (1981), which is a social services report, again confirmed this figure. But then in 1983 the BMA thought there was going to be medical unemployment and called for reducing medical school intake. There was a tremendous outcry from the junior staff, who started conducting surveys to see whether they could find evidence of medical unemployment. In fact, they found only 3 percent unem- ployment over a period of more than three months. A BMA posi- tion paper estimated that by the year 2000 there would need to be at least 9,000 more consultant jobs if there was not going to be great disappointment and failure to meet the expectations of the intake of students.

Only last month, the deans of all the medical schools in the

Figure 15. Applications and Acceptances for Medical Schools, 1983.
Source: UCCA Report, 1982–83.

APPLICATIONS

Home	Men	5182	
	Women	4158	
	Total		9340
Overseas	Men	971	
	Women	418	
	Total		1389
Combined total			10729

ACCEPTANCES

Home	Men	2082	
	Women	1688	
	Total		3770
Overseas	Men	138	
	Women	47	
	Total		185
Combined total			3955

country wrote to *The Times* and said no reduction, please; solve the FMG problem. If you solve the FMG problem, 4,080 annual intake will meet our needs until the end of the century.

Figure 15 shows some interesting data on applications and acceptances to medical schools in England. We had a total of 9,340 applicants from Great Britain and 4,100 (45 percent) were women. We only accept undergraduates in our medical schools from overseas if they come from a country with no medical school. The combined total of applications is 10,729 and the combined acceptances are 3,955.

Another important point is that the number of applicants is falling. It has been as high as 12,000 when there was about a one in three chance of being accepted, but now there is better than a one in three chance of getting into medical school.

Figure 16 shows the state of our problem of finding tenured positions for our registrars. It shows the way the number of junior staff trainees has diverged from the number of consultants, creating an appalling imbalance in which our juniors are in great danger of not being able to fulfill their reasonable expectations. To rectify the imbalance, it has been suggested that the number of consultants should be doubled and the number of registrars should be halved.

Figure 16. Growth in Numbers of Junior Doctors and Consultants: Great Britain, 1970–79. *Source*: House of Commons Report, *Medical Education* (London: Her Majesty's Stationery Office, 1982). Reprinted with permission of the Controller of Her Britannic Majesty's Stationery Office.

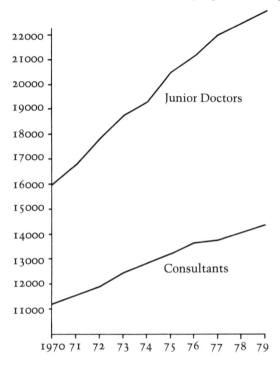

The problem that was recognized in the report from the social services, *Medical Manpower—The Next Twenty Years*,[1] was that the health service in Great Britain is being consultant-led rather than consultant-provided, and consultants are really having much less close contact with patients than they should. The work is being done by an army of juniors who may not have reasonable expectations. The solution is a long way from being found because, although the Department of Health has agreed in principle that the number of consultants should be increased, it is not their job to implement it. Unless they do implement it, we see no solution.

1 Great Britain, Department of Health and Social Security, *Medical Manpower— The Next Twenty Years* (London: Her Majesty's Stationery Office, 1982).

Discussion

DR. RICHARD H. EGDAHL: Two years ago in an area in southeastern Massachusetts, women in Medicaid were unable to get prenatal care because nobody would take care of them; the physicians refused to take them on because the fee did not cover their overhead. So the state worked out something and the local community hospital, at much greater expense, set up clinics for them and the situation blew over. Now it looks as if the state legislature may pass a law that would place a physician's license in jeopardy if he did not take a Medicaid patient. I can see this bill having a real chance of passage. These questions about physicians and where they practice and how they practice and the care of the poor are going to be linked in nettlesome ways as time goes on.

This is the first time I have seen a really serious threat of using the licensure mechanism to insist that a massive cost shifting occur to take care of the unfunded poor.

DR. HARVEY V. FINEBERG: Dr. Anlyan started us on the question, How many doctors do we need? a kind of normative question. This led naturally to consideration of the GMENAC study, which was based on the analysis of need as determined by expert judgment. But we soon shifted focus to the question, How many doctors will be demanded? which is the economic perspective.

We discussed how medical education can respond to the changing social pressures in the population at large and especially in the ideas and attitudes of male and female doctors, the family situation, and so on. We discussed the quality of the pool of medical school applicants and how that can be assured and whether there is or is not a long-term threat to the quality of medical care.

Dr. Tarlov tried to bring us back to a generic question of how to think about the impact or consequences of the growth in supply of physicians without trying to think of it as a question of over- or under-supply. And we discussed how medical school education and the quality of physicians in general can be improved.

The difficulty, of course, is that all these different questions demand very different approaches to thinking about them and to solutions. I feel that it is useful for us to reflect on the question, as Dr. Tarlov posed it, without trying to impose a particular judgment about the numbers. Rather we should think about the consequences of those numbers and which of the consequences have public policy implications, that is, implications that we think might be important for the public.

In thinking of that, I go back to Professor Reinhardt's simple equilibrium of demand and supply. There is an important element in there of price, as in any economic thinking. I believe it is very important for us to be thinking about which of the ways of achieving equilibrium is likely to be the one that will be followed. Will physicians' incomes be adjusted downward? Will the numbers of physicians be adjusted? Or will the demand for services be adjusted? I think those relations are at the heart of the public policy concerns about the future of the supply of physicians.

Once we begin thinking along those lines, it becomes clear that if we talk about the problems from a public perspective of the number and distribution of physicians across specialties and geography we cannot get very far away from thinking about tools like reimbursement systems and other influences on the distribution and the choices that doctors make. In the end these have to be at the heart of trying to deal with the question of doctor supply.

Basically, I think we have to face up to the question about the way doctors are paid. I was very struck with Dr. Graettinger's data about the percentage of first-choice residencies that are not made available to the applicants and how certain of the subspecialties are so popular. That raises a question of whether we have an appropriate mix of choice. Do we want our system of reimbursement or other aspects of reinforcement to lead physicians to certain practice choices? If not, what should we be doing about it? If we are worried about getting services to people in rural or other isolated areas and about making sure that minority groups have an opportunity to pursue careers of their choice, then we ought to deal directly with that policy question.

Although all of these questions are the real policy issues and are, in some sense, incidental to the supply, supply must be a part of the thinking about the solution.

PROFESSOR ROSEMARY A. STEVENS: I think Dr. Fineberg is right that some of the questions relating to income are going to cause all of us great trouble in the next few years.

I would like to suggest two areas where our discussions so far have suggested difficulty. One is conflict arising from within the medical profession and between physicians and nonphysicians; older physicians in conflict with younger physicians; physicians within HMOS and other closed-staff systems being engaged in battles with other people who are not in systems. It is inevitable.

I believe there will also be a male backlash against female physicians. There will certainly be a backlash against foreign medical graduates in the United States. I agree with Dr. Asper that we need to think more about international issues relating to foreign medical graduates.

I think we are going to see competitive conflicts within the specialties among different modalities of care, as well as among well-established specialties. I see tensions coming along, which are part of a perception of a large supply of physicians and the whole question of income levels and expectations.

PROFESSOR JOSEPH P. NEWHOUSE: I would like to second Dr. Fineberg's point. I, too, was struck by Dr. Graettinger's data on the percentage of nonmatches by specialty and its relationship to the perception of excess supply. The same kind of theory I looked at earlier with respect to geographic distribution applies to specialty distribution and suggests that if there is a perception of too many specialties the fee structure is at the bottom of that. My question would be, What exactly determines the fee structure? Is it merely a historical accident that it got to be this way? Does it change over time? If so, what determines this or should there be some intervention in that change? I do not think that the spread of HMOS gets at this particular issue because HMOS have historically been price takers in the market for positions. I think that it is likely to continue to some degree; that is, what HMOS offer will be importantly influenced by incomes that are earned in fee-for-service. Those incomes, in turn, will be influenced by the fee structure. I do think we must address the issue of the fee structure.

DR. ARNOLD S. RELMAN: While I agree entirely with Dr. Fineberg's point that we need to consider the reimbursement of physicians as part of the problem, we should not lose sight of those relatively limited problems of manpower supply that might be dealt with by public policy directed specifically to the supply side. As an example of a limited problem, though a big one, that might be addressed usefully by public policy, I cite the USFMG problem.

The tough issue in this problem is clearly a political one. The state boards, individually, are often under a lot of political pressure to see that the sons and daughters of their constituents who have been educated at Papa Doc universities come back into the system. The overwhelming mass of evidence is that education received at those institutions is grossly inferior. Here we are talking about the possible need of shutting down or reducing the U.S. medical school intake while we allow 4,000 FMGS to come back into the system. While we may not be able to agree on the total number of doctors we need, we all agree that we do not need poorly educated doctors. The question that I raise is, Is there some morally acceptable, legally possible, politically practical way to stop the entrance of 4,000 poorly educated physicians into a pool that many of us feel is getting too large anyway? Is there something that the Federation can do to get the individual state boards off the hook? Is there something that the federal government, through Medicare, can do to get the state boards off the hook? Is there something that the AAMC or the AMA or the LCME can do that takes the political heat off the local legislature so that we can do what is clearly sensible and the right thing? If we really need all those extra students who are going out there to Papa Doc University, we should take them into our own schools. If we do not need them, we should not let them back into the system.

We ought to be fair about it. We ought to "grandfather" them. We ought to say, "Those of you who are out there will have a fair chance to try to get in by passing the examination, but as of a certain date we give you fair warning. Any more of you who start going to Papa Doc U ought to know you are not going to be able to come back into the U.S. system."

MR. JOHN W. COLLOTON: From the perspective of one who deals day to day with the financing of some physician training, I would like to make some comments, not about long-range manpower goals but about some of the immediate financing pressure that teaching hospitals are experiencing and its potential impact on the number of training slots available. Among the 270 teaching hospitals with major college of medicine affiliation there are now some $7 billion of cash flow in what is called the indirect medical education context. The president wants to cut this back by 50 percent in the next fiscal year. There are also some $2 billion of direct medical education expense, which is largely house staff stipend, which the president wishes to freeze. Senator Durenberger wishes to cut back the direct expense by 10 percent and then divert 20 percent of the total now going into graduate medical education into other Medicare initiatives over a span of three or four years.

The business sector, through the PPOs and HMOs, is withdrawing from its traditional involvement in the support of graduate medical education. This may not be because of any philosophical conviction that they should not be involved but rather because under the competitive scheme there is no financing mechanism by which they can pay.

Some of us have the option of going to the states for support, but in Iowa we go to the state facing an uphill struggle: although we are going to ask them to pick up two-thirds of the cost not paid by the federal government, only 35 percent of the products of these programs may remain in the state of Iowa.

The Reagan cuts at the institution I represent would come to $7.2 million in the next fiscal year, including 37 percent of the total direct and indirect educational allowances that we now receive. Therefore what we are doing is sitting down with each clinical department head and addressing the possibility of, first, a 10 percent cut of house staff members and, second, a 20 percent cut. It looks like the department is going to have to control a 10 percent cut through professional fee financing. At 20 percent, they get into the question of cutting back house staff numbers with some subsidy from professional fees.

One must be realistic about where we are in terms of immediate financing of these goals.

MR. EDWIN C. WHITEHEAD: I think perhaps we have omitted another factor that could be rather potent and that is technology. Technology is exerting a very powerful force, and it will increase in power, to reduce the need of physicians, directly and indirectly. I think we are seeing the explosion of self-care, wherein the patient measures his own blood sugars at home and the lady comes to the doctor, not with the question, "Am I pregnant?" but knowing she is pregnant because she did the test at home.

Surgeons are seeing kidney stone crushers that do not need surgeons and microscopy, which is considerably less dramatic and less time consuming, for removing things surgically. There are a number of people who believe that the internist will be using the computer as a tool to help him in his diagnostic techniques and to shorten the amount of time it is necessary to spend with a patient. I think the pathology laboratory is going to disappear as it exists today because it performs a function that is not terribly useful or efficient.

Billions of dollars are going into research by industrial companies for the benefit of the medical community. That research has been guided for the last fifty years by questions of quality: Can we do something a little better? In the past five years, however, the cost element has become far more important. It is a fairly safe assumption that most of the manufacturers of medical equipment and pharmaceuticals are today spending a much greater portion of their assets on cost-improving techniques. Medicine is probably the most labor-intensive industry in our country. We manufacturers are aware that if you want to get a handle on costs, you must reduce labor, and the way to reduce labor is by improvements in technology and techniques. If there is not a physician surplus now, I believe the forces of technology will create a surplus in the not very distant future.

DR. JOSEPH F. BOYLE: There are a couple of things we would all be well advised to keep in mind. As we consider the question of whether or not there are too many physicians or not enough specialists, there is an army out there beginning to do some strange things. They are doing some strange things because of the perceptions that there are too many doctors right now. They are beginning to do funny things because they are being told that there will not be enough work to do. If people persist in this kind of a theme without concrete evidence of the facts, then we may see some doctors doing things we would rather they did not do, because these things are not going to be in the best interest of either the profession or the health of the people.

This is particularly true among younger physicians and medical students who are now in school. They are being told that after having knocked themselves out for virtually a third of their lives to get into medical school, they have made a dumb career choice. They are being advised to look at other options than doing what they went into medical school for in the first place, which was taking care of people.

In each of these instances, we must focus on the question, What is the quality of the medical education experience that is available? We must focus on the quality of care the people are providing. If we look at medical technology, not whether we can do something in a fancier way or a quicker way or more elaborate way but a way that is really going to improve the quality of the service, we can probably do something about containing the costs. We must focus on the available options for people who have an interest in a career in medicine and we must begin mapping out those options and providing some direction to those people. In that way I think we will be doing everybody a far greater service.

Professor Stevens is absolutely correct: these are not all conflicts that will take place in the future; these are conflicts right now. Some of them are getting heated and dangerous among specialties, among physicians, and between physicians and nonphysicians.

We ought to heed Dr. Relman's comments about reducing the number of U.S. graduates while at the same time we let people who go through a truly second-rate school come back here after they graduate. We need to look at how we can assure people of their constitutional right to choose a career and practice it, but subject them to the same kind of evaluation that we have for students who graduate in the U.S. schools without making it more difficult for U.S. graduates to be licensed.

Dr. Galusha and the Federation are to be congratulated for coming along with a means to demonstrate to the public that we are getting serious about licensed physicians being good physicians. We need to tell our state licensing boards to be even more serious than in the past, because the interest of the media in licensing, in discipline, and particularly in cross-state transfers is becoming extremely intense.

Most people going into medicine today expect their incomes to be less. What they need to be told is that there are professional opportunities to pursue a career in which caring for people is the ultimate goal. At the same time, simply saying that you are going to rearrange the way you pay doctors is not going to get people into the inner cities to take care of poor people. They are going to take care of poor people when the opportunity is there to earn a living doing it.

PROFESSOR ELI GINZBERG: First, the federal government is definitely going to try to reduce its flow of money into the system; that is a big flow and it must have an effect upon the behavior of the entire system, including the physicians. Second, the federal government is going to do something about graduate medical education. I don't know whether it will do it this year, next year, or the year following. These are two major developments that we have to begin with.

Dr. Boyle mentioned again the increasing struggle among different sectors of the physician supply that exists today. I think very shortly the state legislatures will hear from disgruntled physicians who feel that they are not as busy as they ought to be.

While I think it is important to do something with FMGs, there are other issues coming up first, because the FMG is such a difficult issue to deal with. I believe we are going to have increasing struggles between new corporate providers—including the old hospitals that are going to be struggling to maintain patients and their physicians who are also going to be struggling to maintain their patients. The conflicts that already exist can only get worse in the face of less money or attempts to control the money. I am by no means sure that less money is going into the system, but I am sure there is going to be an attempt to control the flow of that money.

The important question is, What can the professional leadership do that will make some difference? because otherwise you will still be talking while these issues are being resolved in other ways.

MR. PAUL G. ROGERS: It is interesting that our GMENAC study was based on need, and Dr. Danforth has suggested that it should have been based on demand. Dr. Lister explained that English studies are based on what they can afford. We are beginning to take that perspective here also but not yet in a very significant way. Perhaps some studies should address the question of what we can afford.

As for Dr. Relman's suggestion, I think everyone feels that if our medical schools are going to have to cut down their enrollments, then before we let foreign medical graduates come in and take over they ought to go to those schools. It might well be feasible to work out a national test everyone takes who wants to go to medical school; if they fail that test, they are never to be admitted to any medical school unless they can come back and pass it on a second try. Individual schools could have their own testing over and above that.

It seems that we go through cycles in this country of having a lot of money that we put into all our resources and then having less money when things tighten up. When we have less money we are forced to make critical judgments that we will never face up to otherwise. Maybe this period that we are going through will not be all that bad. We may make judgments that we would never make unless we had to. Maybe this will help us address the foreign medical graduate problem. Maybe this will help us strengthen our whole system to bring forth better doctors and to use them in more effective ways.

DR. ARNOLD S. RELMAN: In a sense the USFMGS took the test that Mr. Rogers suggests they be offered and they flunked it. Almost without exception, USFMGS could not get into any U.S. medical school that they tried to get into, which is not quite the same thing as taking a uniform exam, but they all have had the experience of multiple rejected applications. I am not sure that one could simply decide to take them into the U.S. schools.

MR. PAUL G. ROGERS: If we worked out a system of having those who would go overseas come into the American medical schools instead, we would have to divide 4,000 of them among the 120 U.S. medical schools. That would only be 33 more students per school. If they cannot match up, it seems to me a special course could be set up for them.

DR. JAMES H. SAMMONS: In my view, the financing of medical education is going to have a much greater impact on the numbers of physicians in training than perhaps any other single thing. I hope that we will concentrate on that concern rather than lose our perspective worrying about USFMGS. While Mr. Rogers has expressed some interesting ideas about the USFMG problem, I do not think his solution is politically viable.

Dr. Relman gave us the answer to the question of taking them into our U.S. medical schools: every one of them has had multiple opportunities to be admitted and has failed. The real question is, Are we in a position to do something about the total number of USFMGS? Is it politically, legally possible to do something about it, if we assume that there are too many?

I am concerned that Dr. Fineberg does not understand why the best residencies are the first choices and a very high number of first-choice residencies were not matched. That overlooks the whole process of matching. It does not take into account the people who are program directors in those programs, who had the opportunity to review those individuals before they decided that, for one reason or another, one particular individual was not as suitable for their program as someone else. If you change that process, then you change the numbers. And if you start to change the numbers, then you change the whole thrust of the individual's right to choose his or her special field in medicine. This takes us back very quickly to the problem of who is going to pay for all of these new numbers.

Let us not forget that the only people who think there are too many doctors, according to our survey, are other doctors and the people who are paying the bill, and their solution is to cut the number of doctors so we can reduce the total bill. That might have been true in the past, and it may still be true to a degree, but the changes that are going on today in the form in which medicine is being delivered may substantially affect the total bill, resolving some of those concerns by the payors.

We at the AMA have professional poll takers go into the public once or twice a year with a series of questions that we have been asking for eleven years: Are there too many doctors? Are there not enough doctors? What is the status in your community? What is your opinion?

Almost uniformly the answer comes back: the numbers are essentially correct. Occasionally the public will identify specific specialist needs. Almost routinely, however, certain specialties respond that there are too many, while other specialties respond that there are essentially enough. But the public really does not believe there are too many doctors.

Before we get carried away with this, let us be sure we can meet the expectations that are going to be levied on us by the public: the delivery of care that they perceive is not now being delivered. Whether we or some government agency or some third-party payor thinks it is or not, if there is a perception that there is an unmet need upon the part of the public, then we'd best be very careful how we attempt to manipulate our own system.

DR. TOM E. NESBITT: It is interesting that it costs roughly £3,000 in England to have an operation to remove a kidney stone, but it only costs £800 with the lithotripter. Perhaps technology, when it gets to this country, will really not be all that bad.

I recall Dr. Nicholson telling us there is concern in beginning residency training relating to educational debts, income levels, and expectations of the practice of medicine in the future. Before 1965 physicians could expect four to five times the annual income of union employees. With the advent of Medicare and Medicaid in 1965–66, their income reached eight to nine times what the average hourly wage earner of the unions took home in this country. Taking those yardsticks as having some validity, the profession of medicine can expect to see reductions in annual income. Whether or not those reduced incomes are within the expectation range of college students interested in the profession of medicine is something that needs to be considered.

Ms. Mahoney raises the very valid point that when there is a perception that expectations will not be met in terms of income, some young people with bright minds are going to be turned off. We do not want that; we want to continue to attract the bright minds. I am perfectly comfortable with a physician/population base that is 15 percent of what the expected requirements of our nation might be, but when we come up with other figures that say in fifteen years or twenty years or thirty years that level may be in the range of 50 percent, I am not at all comfortable.

When we talk about the various types of models that we use to try to determine what are reasonable requirements for services, I think it is regrettable that we are not willing to take another look at what an adjusted need-based model might provide us. We struggled long and hard early in GMENAC. We looked at demand-based models that were in existence and we found that they were, in essence, resource driven in terms of money and that they reflected what existed in prior times. We felt that the need-based model, which would reflect the incidence and prevalence of disease and norms of care, could be of some help. We also learned in the analysis of that model that for virtually every specialty there were three or four big-ticket manpower items. If it were possible to follow three or four of those parameters, it would give us some insight into the changes that are occurring in the incidence and prevalence of disease in each of those specialties. With a computerized, mathematical model it could still prove very useful. We should not completely rule that out. The demand-based model, in my view, has not given us a great deal of satisfaction.

DR. ROBERT G. PETERSDORF: I want to comment on the rather narrow point of what California is attempting to do about reducing the number of FMGs in the state. The Bureau of Medical Quality Assurance has set up a number of regulations that specify the curriculum requirements of physicians who practice in the state. For example, they must have seventy-two weeks of clinical experience in the third and fourth year, a certain number of weeks of surgery, and so on. Many graduates of offshore medical schools cannot meet those requirements and this was, of course, the purpose of the exercise. However, it has backfired on us in a major way because virtually no member of an M.D./Ph.D. program can meet those requirements. Characteristically, these people have truncated clinical experiences, especially in surgery. People from outside the state whose medical schools did not have the same kind of curricular requirement also are unable to meet the licensing requirements.

The reason the Bureau of Medical Quality Assurance went through this exercise was to be fair to everybody. Because they did not want to get sued, they laid the same requirements on the graduates of LCME-accredited schools as they did on non-LCME-accredited schools. This created a lot of turmoil among program directors who are choosing interns and also among young physicians who want to come to California to intern and to take their residency training.

I believe that the purpose of the Bureau of Medical Quality Assurance was laudable but they failed to think it through and they did not interpret it well. Before you go through this exercise at your state level, design it very carefully lest it hurt the graduates of U.S. schools as much as it keeps the FMGs out.

DR. JOHN E. AFFELDT: Dr. Lister brought to our attention the difference between the open system in the United States and the closed system in Great Britain. I think we are beginning to see the open system in the United States close a little bit. I do not anticipate that it is going to close completely, but we certainly can see some closure occurring, particularly in medical staff membership. One area of conflict which I think will increase is clinical privileges, that is, the hospital delineating clinical privileges. We are beginning to hear the term "economic profile" of a physician emerge instead of competency profile. That will be yet another area of conflict.

MS. MARGARET MAHONEY: The thinking of Clark Kerr on the Carnegie Commission fifteen years ago was not unlike the thinking of Eli Ginzberg today. If it is any comfort, the situation did not look very different fifteen years ago than it looks today. The questions were to some degree the same, although they were reversed on the issue of how many physicians we needed. After doing some very careful economic analyses of manpower issues, from which he learned about the maldistribution of physicians, Clark Kerr was led to say that he was going to take two particular issues —quality and maldistribution—and build around them a framework in which he could develop an agenda. That agenda included the development of new schools, the concept of AHEC, and a number of other very carefully delineated steps, because Kerr believed strongly that he would like to let the market take care of some of the problems.

We are pretty much in that same position today although one additional problem today is that some principles are in jeopardy. Some human conflicts we see are the result of people's freedom of choice being questioned. We cannot hit at the FMGS squarely, but I think we can find some devices once we say what we would like to hit.

DR. ALVIN R. TARLOV: Given that there will be an increase in supply of physicians and the needs of the patient population are not going to grow as fast, then we are likely to see a continuation in the erosion of the number of patients seen by each doctor. Perhaps the leadership of the medical profession ought to be discussing with the profession how it can best use that freed-up time. The options seem to fall into a couple of categories. Doctors can elect to have more leisure time. Perhaps physicians would take more time for conversation with their patients about such issues as health promotion or their disease or their drugs or counseling of other sorts. Maybe we could return to the time when physicians, as part of their creed, devoted a certain amount of their time to the unfortunate in society who had no access to medical care, or who today have no insurance. Perhaps some physicians might elect to devote part of their time to providing some kind of care and public health services in Third World countries.

DR. EUGENE S. MAYER: I think that a good number of private physicians in North Carolina are telling their state legislators that we have enough physicians here. These words are falling on deaf ears for two reasons. One is that there still are communities where citizens are telling legislators that they have unmet needs. Second, and perhaps more important, there are some people who are telling legislators that while we may be approaching a surplus or a sufficiency, if they cut opportunities for medical education in North Carolina, people are simply going to come into this state who are poorly trained at less desirable medical schools outside the country. Once those points are made, we find a rapid dissipation of interest in the legislature. Regardless of what should or should not be done with the U.S. medical school graduates, my prediction would be that legislators are going to have a hard time cutting medical school class sizes at home, which clearly are opportunities for sons and daughters in the state.

DR. DANIEL C. TOSTESON: It seems quite clear that everyone agrees more or less about how many doctors there are going to be. The problem is on the side of how many do we need, demand, want, desire. Both epidemiological and economic models seem unable to answer that question.

Very hard to predict in this complicated scene in which we are now living and are going to be living is how many would be employed? This is made harder to determine because it is not clear who will be buying their services, corporate employers or individuals. To my mind, this confusion goes to a central question that has to do with the very roots of the profession.

Let me cast it by contrasting the medical industry, as it has emerged, with the medical profession. Professions arise when buyers cannot be prudent about advice. We cannot expect ordinary citizens to choose medical services without advice. Doctors presumably help them in that manner. It seems to me that that advisory role, the role of a professional, contrasts very sharply with the innumerable roles of physicians as employees in the rising medical industry. Until we in the profession think through clearly in our own minds how much we want to continue to be a profession, as compared with experts in a complicated industry, we are going to find it difficult to estimate how many people we need in the field.

When I think about what is going to be happening to the graduates of our medical schools, it is perfectly obvious to me that most of them are going to be employed in one or another segment of this complicated industry. What is not at all clear to me is how many are going to be performing the traditional roles of physicians. This makes the designing of educational strategies problematic in the extreme.

DR. WILLIAM H. DANFORTH: University education really did not come up until Dr. Tosteson's comment, I think not because it is not important, not because it is not difficult to plan a good university, including medical school education, but because what goes on inside our institutions is being affected by, rather than affecting, the external environment we are all so concerned about.

One area of conflict that I expect is between scientific medicine and more bizarre forms of medicine. As some of our bright students graduate, if they cannot make the kind of living they want following what they have been taught in medical school, they may invent some other ways of making a living.

Another important area that could lead to conflict is attempting to take the indirect cost of medical education or the direct cost of graduate education out of the health care dollar. I can see nothing but problems coming out of that effort. It seems to me that if we wanted to single out one thing we would like to stop, it would be that effort. There is really no logical reason why graduate education or medical education should not come out of the health care dollar. Graduate education of other kinds comes out of consumer dollars. Training programs in industry are paid for by consumer dollars; training programs in large industries that are major government suppliers, such as industries that supply the military, have training programs which can be charged.

DR. JOHN S. GRAETTINGER: First, how many doctors do we need and for what? I have not quite heard an answer yet, but certainly graduate medical education, not undergraduate education, is where the answer is. Second, how important are the aspirations of students? I am distressed when I see a quarter of those who want training in obstetrics and gynecology not getting a post. I don't know whether that is important or not, but I think it needs to be addressed when we are talking about needs.

We have so far discussed only the surplus side of need. Are there any shortage areas left? Are we still short possibly of psychiatrists? If so, why? Do we have needs in any shortage areas? And, finally, why do we have more graduate medical education positions than are needed for the graduate medical education of our U.S. seniors? Clearly they reflect funded service needs as a component of residency training. I am still concerned about that vacuum that inexorably leads to some four thousand more physicians annually than any of us seem to want.

DR. BRYANT L. GALUSHA: I think we all know what we have: we have an enviable medical educational system. We have an enviable health care delivery system in this country which is being assaulted. We have supply problems, cost problems, specialty distribution problems, and geographic distribution problems.

One problem that worries me today is the enormity of the pool of physicians that are being backlogged. What will happen to them? What problems will emerge out of that pool? I do not know the answer to that, nor do I know how to address it, but I think it is something that we should address here.

DR. JOHN LISTER: One of the major achievements of the NHS is that we have managed to get a much more even distribution of physicians, both primary care and specialists, throughout the country. The general practitioners' services, administered by family practitioner committees, may exert a kind of negative direction of labor because they only allow people to go into an area if there is a need on the basis of doctors per population.

Hospital services are regionalized and the regional health authorities have done a great deal to improve the services in their regions. In the early stages there was a great expansion in the number of young consultants who were appointed. There was a working party some years ago called the Resource Allocation Working Party which brought about a redistribution of resources throughout the country and the regions which enabled them to upgrade services. One of the reasons why we are economical on specialists is that there are regional centers; neurosurgery, cardiothoracic surgery, nephrology, and radiotherapy are very often regionally based.

Dr. Danforth mentioned the question of who should fund graduate education. This, of course, is another good thing about the National Health Service. The National Health Service recognizes that it must fund the continuing education of the doctors in the service.

3

Public and Private Options for Assessing and Managing Physician Manpower Supply

ROBERT G. PETERSDORF, M.D.

I begin with the assumption that the evidence is mounting that we have too many physicians in this country. I want to concentrate on part of the pipeline that feeds the system, namely, the house staff. I will begin with the contention that the house staff is too large.

What is the evidence for this? Over a decade ago, the SOSSUS study pointed out that there were too many surgeons, both in practice and in training. Surgery chose to handle this issue by declaring that too many non-board-certified surgeons were doing surgery and by suggesting that if those people would stop operating, surgical training programs would not have to be cut. Of course the general practitioners did not quit operating and while the training programs in surgery have not increased, they have not decreased.

Then came the Study of Internal Medicine Manpower, which did not necessarily prove that there were too many internists, but showed beyond a doubt that following a three-year training program in general internal medicine, close to 70 percent of fully trained internists obtained further training in and then practiced a subspecialty. The subspecialists in medicine have been multiplying like rabbits and everyone now agrees that there are too many of them. Yet, despite this consensus, there is no decrease in the number of trainees in the subspecialties of internal medicine. The reason, apparently, is that the replication of the race is the life blood of most training program directors, a goal in which they are aided and abetted by two charter academic right-to-life organizations, the American Board of Internal Medicine and the American College of Physicians.

Next came GMENAC, the report which has been attacked from every angle, depending on whose ox was being gored. GMENAC may not be quantitatively entirely accurate, but qualitatively it is almost surely correct. Evidence for this is seen both in the world of private practice where good positions in the subspecialties are getting harder and harder to find and in the world of academe where we are seeing progressively greater competition from the very trainees of whom we were once so proud. Yet despite this competition and the lack of referrals that accompanies it, we continue to train subspecialists, using the arguments that if we do not train them somebody else will.

The most convincing data indicating a surfeit of specialty trainees are as follows: 13,221 (18.3 percent) of our house staff were FMGS on September 1, 1983. It seems fair to ask at this point whether the large number of FMGS whom we are training is necessarily bad. The answer has to be a resounding yes, because the medical background most of these trainees bring from their medical schools to their training programs is appallingly poor.

It is claimed that the basic science teaching at the medical school in Grenada, for instance, is pretty good and that most students pass the national boards. In fairness, St. George's in Grenada is probably the best of the lot. The same cannot be said for many schools in Dominica, Mexico, and elsewhere in which conditions for the students are nothing short of deplorable. These, then, are the house staff with which we are still populating nearly 20 percent of our internship and residency positions—many of which have no reason for existing.

Unfortunately, the problem of the foreign medical graduates is not improving. Many FMGS continue to enter this country, often on nonvisitor visas. While no direct figures on foreign matriculants are available, several indirect measures provide some assessment of the magnitude of this problem. Of the number of U.S. citizens who have graduated from foreign medical schools, those seeking certification to enter graduate medical education in this country rose from 860 in 1974 to 2,800 in 1982. In 1982, 1,037 American nationals who were then enrolled in foreign medical schools sought advanced standing in U.S. schools; 826 of these came from seven proprietary schools located in Mexico and the Caribbean. A 1980 GAO report estimated the enrollment of American nationals in foreign medical schools to be between 8,000 and 11,000.

If the evidence that the house staff is too large is convincing, what options do we have? The cuts should occur first of all in the FMG positions. Many of the house staff programs that are populated predominantly by FMGs are second and third rate and are on and off probation. Although it is difficult to discontinue poor residency programs, many of the 13,000 FMG house officers and the programs at which they train could be phased out without seriously compromising the quality of graduate medical education in this country.

Even accredited programs are often too large. I know of very few training programs that have shrunk—most have grown. So-called educational requirements also contribute to increasing the size of house staff. For example, neurology trainees must put in time in neuropathology, neuroradiology, and sometimes even neurosurgery. In order to fulfill these educational requirements, more house staff must be hired and paid. I agree entirely with the recent pronouncement of the AAMC that the financial impact of changes in house staff programs should be assessed by an impartial body before specialty boards mandate changes in residency requirements. However, the AAMC's plea to the ABMS that something be done about this seems to have fallen on deaf ears.

Another reason for large house staff programs is that today's residents do not want to work as hard as those of us who belonged to the generation of iron house officers that I did. They do not want to work as many nights and they want more vacation and, in order to accede to these requests, there have to be more house staff. The desire of both house staff and faculty to have exposure to different specialties and subspecialties adds to the number of residents required. Suffice it to say that the number of residents has grown much more rapidly than the number of medical students.

If it is true that the house staff is too large, let us review some options for reducing its size. The first is voluntary; I am too old and cynical to believe that this will work. Second, it is possible to mandate reduced house staff positions legislatively at the state and federal levels. The University of California has been mandated by the legislature to reduce the number of residents under its aegis by several hundred. However, this reduction is more apparent than real, because most of the resident positions are being reduced in hospitals affiliated with the university. In order to comply with this legislative mandate, the university will simply disaffiliate from those hospitals whose residency programs will continue, unchanged in size, as unaffiliated programs. At the federal level, one version of the Durenberger Bill reduces funding for reimbursement of residents by 10 percent. Unless the hospitals find a different source of funding, this is tantamount to a legislative reduction in the number of residents.

Third, there are the specialty boards. Many of these, notably the American Board of Internal Medicine, do not think that they should correct physician manpower supply through board requirements. The ABIM can claim credit for the increase in the number of medical specialties by having instituted subspecialty boards in ten of the subspecialties of internal medicine. Another board has floated the proposal that it would not admit to its examinations graduates of foreign medical schools. Aside from the fact that this would probably not stand up in court, it is a way of reducing the role of foreign medical graduates in that particular specialty.

I believe that board requirements can be made stiffer by requiring either longer periods of training or longer periods of practice in the specialty before permitting an individual access to specialty examination. It can be safely predicted that the number of individuals opting for subspecialties will decrease, although probably not steeply, the longer the time period between training and the examination.

Fourth, stiffer accreditation requirements could be adopted. Many residency review committees demand that residency programs provide trainees with sufficient clinical contact in terms of both the number of patients seen and the number of procedures performed. If all accreditation requirements could be stiffened somewhat, a number of training programs would fall by the wayside because the clinical material for training would not be available. Part of this is a direct consequence of the over-training of subspecialists who have taken patients to community hospitals and out of the aegis of university training programs.

Fifth, incentives could be made available to hospitals that voluntarily reduce the size of their training programs. For example, if the government chose to match training funds saved by the hospital, the hospital could build up a nice nest egg and use these funds to purchase equipment, repair its physical plant, and institute new programs.

Much has been written about the fact that the number of house staff cannot be cut without cutting medical school class size. While medical student class size has to be cut eventually, the fact is that in the intermediate term we have far more house officers than medical students. Medical school output can be decreased in one of two ways. One, a number of medical schools, particularly in states that have created one or more new schools during the past decade, could be closed. Second, the number of students in each medical school can be reduced by a sizable number. There are, however, several countervailing forces to this tactic. The first and most important is access. Although the ratio of applicants to acceptances to medical school dropped from 3:1 in 1974 to 2:1 in 1984, there is little evidence that the quality of the applicants has dropped sharply. Moreover, how can a legislator withstand the pressure from the disgruntled constituent, whose offspring, with a 3.5 grade point average, has not been accepted by the state school, which is supported by that constituent's tax dollar, and who now has to go to a private Eastern medical school or, worse still, an offshore school at many times the cost?

The schools themselves are ambivalent about decreasing class size because state schools often lose resources if they decrease class size, while in private schools high tuitions make money at the margin. The schools also argue that if they decrease class size it would only lead to more students going to Grenada, Guadalajara, and Dominica. What is the value in letting poorly trained students loose on the country at the expense of well-trained ones?

Physician manpower can, of course, be controlled by simply withholding reimbursement for groups of trainees that are in surplus. These might include foreign medical graduates or specialties that are declared to be in surplus, based on available manpower studies. Hospitals would simply not be reimbursed for house staff in those categories. Conversely, shortage specialties could be encouraged by direct subsidies to hospitals. A national health manpower commission would be needed to implement such a program if it were administered at the national level or a statewide commission if such a program were commissioned at the state level. This is probably the only option that I have mentioned so far with enough teeth in it to work.

A recent report of the inspector general has suggested that house staff stipends be paid out of professional fees after only the first year of training. The report further argues that the professional fee charged and paid to the combination of house officer and attending should not exceed that paid to an attending working without house staff in a community hospital. While not aimed directly at reducing the number of trainees, it almost certainly will do just that because neither full-time nor part-time faculty would be willing to share their professional fees with house staff, except in very unusual circumstances.

Let me present a plan that will address two issues: one, the excessive size of the house staff, and two, its excessive costs that put the teaching hospital at a competitive disadvantage with the community hospital. The plan makes the basic assumption that we have a social contract to provide every graduate of an American LCME-accredited medical school with three years of house staff training. That enables the individuals in the specialties of family practice, pediatrics, and internal medicine to fulfill basic primary care board requirements.

We presently have 72,000 house officers in this country, 13,000 of whom are foreign medical graduates. I would like to convince you that a large number of these FMGS have to be eliminated from the pool, which would leave 59,000 house officers. We have about 18,000 U.S. graduates annually or 54,000 every three years. This leads to the fact that we would have to eliminate 5,000 house officers—the difference between today's 59,000 U.S. graduate house officers and the plan's 54,000—which is somewhere under 10 percent. Now, what should the specialty distribution of these 54,000 house officers be? Let us assume that a surplus of primary care physicians is less deleterious than a surplus of specialists. Let us also assume an ideal ratio of primary care physician to specialist to be 70:30.

The primary care doctors would then be 70 percent of the 54,000 or 37,800. As figure 17 shows, half of these should go into internal medicine and a significant number into family medicine, pediatrics, and obstetrics. The remaining 30 percent go into the specialties, divided equally among surgery, the several specialties of anesthesiology, radiology, and pathology, and the remainder, which are mainly neurosciences and psychiatry.

Figure 17. Specialty Distribution.

70% PRIMARY CARE	37,800
Internal medicine	18,900
Family medicine	7,600
Pediatrics	6,500
Ob/Gyn	4,800
30% SPECIALTIES	16,200
Surgery & surgery specialties	5,400
Anesthesiology, radiology, pathology	5,400
Remainder	5,400

Figure 18. Percentage of Residents by Specialty, 1983.

Residency	Percent	Cumulative
Internal medicine	24.3%	24.3%
General medicine	10.9	35.2
Family practice	10.0	45.2
Pediatrics	8.5	53.7
Ob/Gyn	6.4	60.1
All others	39.9	100.0

Figure 18 shows the percentages of residents by specialty in 1983. If you take the present house staff in training in internal medicine, family practice, pediatrics, and obstetrics, they account, at least at the entry point, for 50 percent. We are going to try to shift that to 70 percent by a major downsizing in the specialties of surgery, pathology, radiology, and anesthesiology.

For the purpose of financing this plan, I will postulate that house officers are students and should not be funded from patient revenues. Of a number of alternatives, the creation of a general medical education fund derived from either tax revenues or an all-payor surcharge and based on a per capita funding of house officers seems a fair way to go. The fund should be relatively easy to administer and, for the sake of argument, an average stipend should be $24,000. I also suggest an indirect education cost of 18 percent and a 2 percent cost for administering the program. In total, that cuts the house staff bill by about a third. Salaries decline from $1.7 billion, according to the latest data given by the AAMC, to $1.3 billion. Fringe benefits remain the same at 15 percent but decline in dollars from $255,000 to $195,000. The indirect costs decrease from 40 percent to 18 percent, so the total bill declines by $880 million, from $2.6 billion to $1.75 billion.

I believe fundamentally in internal autonomy, and we must not necessarily say that we need only house officers who get three years of training. Rather, we *pay* for three years of training. If house officers need to train longer or if people in internal medicine want fellows, they must find other ways to pay for them. At the University of Washington, I put no hospital or departmental money into specialty training and we had 140 fellows; this attests to the great ingenuity of division heads in gathering money.

What are the possible sources for funding additional training? First, there are professional fees. If, for example, a pulmonary fellow sees a patient before the attending sees him, that fellow is saving the attending a great deal of time. Why not pay the fellow part of the fee? Second, some hospitals have endowments bearing gifts. Third, the medical school could pay something to house officers for the role they play in teaching medical students. They are, after all, graduate assistants. The graduate assistant in anthropology gets a small stipend from the university; why shouldn't the medical school pay the hospital a small stipend for helping to train our medical students?

There would be two mechanisms for shoring up shortage specialties, either special opportunity grants from the government or an overall manpower commission to run this kind of program.

While the program I describe might set up yet another bureaucratic colossus, I hope it would not. I would propose that every hospital with a training program must become affiliated with a medical school. That school, in concert with the hospitals, will determine whether a given hospital should have a training program, in what specialties such a program should exist, and how many trainees there should be in each program. In other words, I am resurrecting the doctrine of institutional responsibility that was postulated by the educational establishment at least ten years ago.

The general medical education fund would be distributed by the Bureau of Health Manpower to a fiscal intermediary—I would suggest the AAMC—and it in turn would give the money to the medical schools or the hospitals. The Bureau of Health Manpower would have a manpower advisory council that would set policy and determine whether and when changes in the percentage of trainees in various specialties should occur. Such changes should be mandated no more often than once a year and perhaps no more often than every three years. In order to stimulate shortage specialties, the bureau could set the numbers at a different level and sponsor a program of special opportunity grants. Any program that mandates this degree of change would require a long phase-in period, and I suggest beginning the program in 1988 since it very likely would require some degree of federal regulation.

This program permits a good deal of free choice for the medical schools and their teaching hospitals. It employs a private agency to administer it and turns to the federal government only for the money, for overall physician manpower policy, and for the administration of a modest-sized grant program.

Let me address briefly some objections to this plan that have been raised. The first is to the use of federal dollars and the political pressures that this might bring. I counter by saying that the country's future physician pool is a national resource and thus should be everybody's obligation. The question can also be raised why the onus for financing house staff training should be placed on the federal government rather than the states. I have seen enough state legislatures play havoc with medical education and I think we would get more equity if we had the federal government do it.

The next major objection is why the federal government should subsidize physicians who are likely to have high incomes in the future. First, it seems unlikely that these high incomes will persist. Second, many physicians now entering practice are $100,000 or so in debt. Finally, those who enter a surplus, high-earning specialty can always be given their house staff stipends in the form of loans; then a payback system can be devised to forgive the loans, to forgive the interest on the loans, or to charge the full interest, as the case may be.

One of the virtues of this program is that all the educational costs would be removed from the hospital reimbursement formula. In a price-competitive environment, the teaching hospital would be able to compete on the basis of its efficiency and the quality of its service and not use educational costs as an excuse for its higher prices.

Neither this nor any other plan should be set in concrete. Already many modifications have been suggested, including full funding for primary board certification, a salary scale for different levels of residency training, and modifications in the FMG formula. No matter what is done, we need to keep in mind that the excess number of house officers coming out of the training pipeline are at the base of the physician surplus.

In conclusion, I hope we can agree on the following: specialty maldistribution of physicians is not being addressed by market-place forces and we need to do something about it; graduate medical education is too bloated and too expensive; and any plan that alters the system must benefit not only the teaching hospitals, their faculties and their trainees, but also society in general.

Unless we devise some reforms to address these issues, we will almost surely bring down upon ourselves more draconian measures that will destroy our present system of graduate medical education, and if that happens we will have nobody to blame but ourselves.

Comments

I. From the AAMC

JOHN A. D. COOPER, M.D.

It is clear that there is widespread concern that we may have or will have too many physicians to provide the amount of care that policymakers from government, business, labor, and the insurance industry believe we can afford. However, some people are concerned about the accessibility of medical care and among those who have this concern are legislators at both the state and national levels who do not agree that we have too many physicians to meet the demands for care in this country.

There are really two ways of deciding how many physicians one should have. First, one could argue that, within the limits of the resources available for quality education programs, one should provide a place for every qualified student who wishes to study medicine. This is the way universities treat all their educational programs except medicine. They do not decide that there are not enough jobs for Greek professors or Greek graduates and then cut back on the number of students who want to major in Greek. If you want to major in Greek and are qualified to get in the program, you can major in Greek. This approach is warmly supported by those who wish to become physicians and by parents who want their sons and daughters to become physicians. As a matter of fact, in 1968 the Association of American Medical Colleges and the American Medical Association adopted a policy which said that a place should be provided for every qualified student who wishes to study medicine. To my knowledge, neither organization has rescinded, withdrawn, or modified that position statement.

Second, one could decree that the number of places in medical schools should be related to the number of physicians needed by the medical care system. One of the problems with this approach is how to make the decision about the number of physicians we need, particularly during a period of very rapid change in the content and the organization of medical practice. Should the decision be made by the president of the United States? Should it be made by the Congress? Should it be made by the secretary of health and human services? Should it be made by HCFA? Should it be made by the National Association of Manufacturers? By the AFL-CIO? By state government? By the AMA or the AHA or the AAMC? Who will make the decision and upon what basis? It is very clear that in this country, as well as in other countries, the decision of how many physicians we have is really a political decision which depends upon the view of the policymakers as to what fraction of our wealth we wish to devote to medical care.

I would like to point out something about the GMENAC study and its conclusions. If one examines that study, one finds that it predicts that we will have 12 percent more physicians in the year 1990 than the study recommends as the need-based number of physicians. I think we have done a darn good job.

Think back thirty years, because that is the period over which physicians now in practice have been prepared, educated, and trained. Think about what has happened in medicine over those thirty years. There has been a revolution in the content of medicine, in the armamentarium of the physician, and in the procedures and the technology of medicine. There has been a revolution in accessibility to medical care. In spite of all that really remarkable change in medicine, we came out—without any of these predictors or people telling us how many physicians we should or should not have—within 12 percent of what was determined to be the optimal number. I seriously doubt that anybody could have predicted as accurately over these years the number of physicians we would have needed or even the number within certain types of specialties.

I am reminded of Eli Ginzberg's story about being asked by the governor of New York to make a study in the middle forties about how many beds they needed for tuberculosis patients and how many pulmonary physicians ought to be trained. Eli, in his usual manner, developed a group, studied all of this, and came back to tell the governor they needed to double the number of tuberculosis beds and double the number of pulmonary physicians being trained to cover the needs of the tuberculosis patients. Within two years they were decreasing the hospital beds set aside for tuberculosis patients, and pulmonary physicians were having a hard time staying busy because streptomycin and isoniazid had been discovered.

Sometimes one wonders how much we should depend upon

soothsayers' predictions in areas where there is very rapid change. I think we can argue that market forces have indeed been pretty effective over the past three decades.

As far as numbers go, U.S. medical schools are no longer the gatekeepers of the number of physicians in practice in the United States. We have gone through the litany of how many foreign medical graduates—aliens and U.S. citizens—are coming to or returning to this country, and I think one could argue that if these people are going to attend medical school and come here and go into practice, although we may be able to keep them out, it would be better to have them trained in a good school than in any one of the schools in the Caribbean. I think that if we reduce class size we will just give a stimulus to those Caribbean entrepreneurs to open up more schools and expand the ones they have. The national associations really do not have the power to direct their constituencies to change their class sizes or even the mix of residencies that are related to the institutions. All we can do is make sure the quality of education is maintained and the number of institutions giving education and the number of students we educate are related to the resources that are available.

When state schools start to cut back on class size, their legislature starts to cut funding. The private schools lose the marginal gains from the tuition of the students they cut out; even though this is a very small amount of money, it still is a very important part of their unrestricted income. The problem is that the resources of an academic medical center are only to a small extent related to the education and training of the medical students. The academic medical center is a multipurpose institution that is doing much more than educating medical students. Society may not want it reduced on the basis of these other contributions it is making. The Board of Regents of the State of Ohio tried to close the medical schools—I think one might argue that there are too many medical schools in Ohio—but they were unable to, not because the people in those communities where the medical schools are located are concerned about the numbers of medical students they are educating and training but because of what those institutions have done to raise the quality of care and to expand the accessibility of that kind of care to the citizens in those communities.

II. From the AMA

JAMES H. SAMMONS, M.D.

The AMA positions are always subject to change based on the actions of the House of Delegates, but up to this point we do not believe there is a surplus of physicians nor are we in favor of artificial efforts to manipulate the system. We do believe that the free enterprise market economy is going to have an impact and is beginning to show evidence of that already. We do believe that competition is clearly there and getting stiffer every minute and that that, too, will affect the system. We would oppose vigorously federal intervention by setting artificial quotas. We would oppose very vigorously state interventions to artificially set quotas.

We do believe it is the responsibility of each university to appropriately and intelligently decide for itself what portion of its resources will be devoted to medical education and the size of its own student body.

Having said all that, let me go back and review with you some of the things I think may very well be happening and some of the things we ought maybe to be doing, not because we want to change class size but simply because they need to be done in the first place for quality purposes.

One can argue forever about the numbers and the ratios. GMENAC has been a favorite whipping boy for people who disagreed with it and it has been the podium for people who agreed with it. I propose to do neither except to say that, if nothing else, it at least gives an excellent position from which one can debate the issues. We do not agree that there are too many physicians nor do we agree that the ratios are wrong. Our multiple lawyers are very concerned that we not give the impression of attempting to artificially manipulate the numbers.

I have heard several people suggest that the residency review committees are not enforcing quality review to the degree that they should. Since the AMA is a member of every residency review committee, I am going to see to it that our people take a very different approach to the question of the essentials for accreditation and that they attempt to improve that quality. Maybe that will reduce the number of positions, perhaps the two thousand positions that Dr. Petersdorf said would be excess if you eliminated portions of the medical population. Whether it will or not remains to be seen, but it is clearly something we ought to be doing anyway, even if it only reduces by one.

It is our opinion, as Mr. Colloton so beautifully pointed out, that hospital budgets and reimbursement methodologies for patient care are going to have a quicker and stronger impact on the entire supply problem than any of us could have, even if we all agreed that we wanted some sort of legislative approach. I am not sure that is all good. Whether you agree or disagree that residents are totally learning or totally giving care or somewhere in the middle is immaterial; the fact of the matter is, many hospital settings and a great many people would be sorely displaced if we suddenly and arbitrarily removed residents from their locus at this point in history. There is no available mechanism to soak up the need for that patient care.

There is no question of competition beginning; it is out there already. Competition is going to affect doctors' income and their ability to maintain a practice. Competition among ourselves may be the finest competition in the world because it can be based not only on price but on quality of care, on ability, and on training. The competition that bothers me is outside of medicine, among paramedicals that are springing up all over the place. I have yet to see the universities arbitrarily, capriciously, or even carefully and deliberately decide that they will close some of their training programs in paramedical areas. I have not seen any of them decide that they are producing too many technicians.

I have not seen anybody yet take the position that in order to stabilize the system we have to reduce the outside competitors for the inside quality of medicine. It would be interesting to see a university face up to that, since so many of them now are willing to face up to the fact that their teaching hospitals are drags on their budgets, that they simply cannot afford to keep them, that they have to sell them, to divest themselves in some fashion because the hospital is impairing their ability to maintain the rest of the university.

Finally, we have the third group—the limited licensed practitioners, who are becoming more troublesome and more dangerous. They are grabbing onto larger and larger pieces of medical care and, in my personal opinion, are becoming less qualified to have what they presently have. They constitute another big area of competition in medicine today that will ultimately have a substantial impact on the ability of physicians to maintain their practices.

How do we resolve these problems? Maybe we ought to tighten up the admission requirements, not because we want to limit the numbers but because there may be something wrong with the admission requirements. I personally take the position that what we have done is allow computers to decide who is and who is not going to be a physician because we let the computer make the first cut. If we are going to tighten up admission requirements, let us not only tighten them up for admission to medical school, let us also tighten them up from the standpoint of getting a license to practice. Let us not allow political influence to determine who does and does not get a license to practice from the state boards. Let us strengthen the state boards, finance them differently, give them more investigators, and then stand behind them when they refuse to issue a license.

If a change in the law is needed, it should say that someone whose license has just been revoked cannot run down to the local courthouse, get it back, and then spend five or six years stalling the case while continuing to practice. Maybe we should be making that change anyway, regardless of the number of doctors.

The suggestion has been made that we can solve some of this problem by lengthening the residency program. I wonder if that is really true. Is that really going to reduce the number of residents in any given program or is it just a one-time shot that will have no further impact two years later because the first year of lengthening will still not avoid the entrance of the first year of additional people into the program? I really do not think that pathologists downstream are going to find that they have substantially reduced the number of pathologists simply by adding another year to the training program.

The FMG problem is almost insurmountable. There is almost no way that you can justify unusual and arbitrary limits on U.S. citizens. We would agree that there should be absolutely no differentiation between the examinations and the qualifications for those people who come home to practice and for those people who stay at home and attempt to go into practice. I would have a great deal of difficulty with the concept that U.S. citizens could be denied their right to return home and pursue their chosen field simply because they did not stay here. I would be equally opposed to giving them any kind of unusual advantage not given to the students here.

Over the next few years I think we will see some impact on the number of doctors in this country simply because the economics of the situation are going to demand it. I think we are seeing that now. There has to be a reason why 2.8 applicants per admission has declined to 2. There is nothing different about medicine, except that it is more exciting, more viable, and has a greater future than ever before. Yet the number of applicants is decreasing. Clearly, the economic realities of medicine are not escaping the notice of student bodies in undergraduate universities in this country.

Vertical integration, which is my choice of words for what I believe is going to happen over the next five to ten years in the delivery of health care in this country, is going to affect the number of people who want to go into this profession.

I simply repeat that the AMA does not believe that there is an excess, nor would we agree to either the federal or state govenment intervening in the arbitrary determination of quotas of entry into the medical schools or into specialties of medicine.

III. From a Private Medical School[1]

DANIEL C. TOSTESON, M.D.

I think we know pretty well how many doctors there are going to be in the year 2000 and we know pretty well what the total population of this country will be in the year 2000. What we do not know is how many doctors we are going to need, require, demand, or desire. There seems to be general agreement that the economic rather than the epidemiological model is the way to address that question.

I suppose the bottom line in the numbers game in terms of response from private schools is, What do you intend to do with your class size? I do not think that private medical schools should reduce class size in order to regulate the number of people entering into medicine. I do not think that medical schools generally, and certainly not private medical schools, should take upon themselves that kind of regulatory function. It may very well be that some private medical schools will wish to reduce class size. I hope that when they do this they will do so on the basis of the quality of the education.

The function of medical schools as components of universities

1 Presented in part at the "Conference on the Investor-Related Academic Health Center and Medical Education," held in Phoenix, Arizona, on February 21, 1985, and sponsored by the AMA, the AHA, and the AAMC.

is to prepare for the medicine of tomorrow; that means people and ideas. I think we should assess our performance in terms of how well we are doing that job. If we are not doing it well enough because we have too many students, then we should reduce the number of students, but it should be only for that reason that we reduce class size.

Perhaps one other reason that I would mention for not reducing class size is this: we all know that in the research-oriented academic medical centers undergraduate medical education is a marginal activity from the point of view of expenditures, maybe encompassing 5 percent of the total activity of these institutions. To make it even more marginal would seem to me to be sending the wrong kind of signal with regard to the importance of this social function.

Let me now discuss a couple of directions for change. First, the rise of corporate medicine. This comes from scientific discoveries, technological inventions, and new procedures and new facilities, all making the industry of medicine rise in parallel with and in some ways swamp the profession of medicine. The rise of corporate medicine has created or is expressed by a series of more complicated organizations delivering care. Corporate medicine is changing the roles that physicians play. More often, physicians are employees; often they are functioning as technical experts on some large team. Even in our teaching hospitals, frequently it is hard to find someone who will sit down with a worried patient or parent and explain what is going on.

Physicians function in a complex way economically. They function as a buyer for the patient and, increasingly in corporate medicine, they are marketing the services of the corporation. They have competing allegiances, to patients as professionals and to corporations as employees. In short, corporate medicine is heightening the conflict between medical and financial incentives for physicians, and this to my mind moves them from a doctor/patient relationship in the traditional sense to a much more complex set of relationships.

These changes in physicians' roles are changing the goals for medical education. We need in our private as well as public medical schools to be thinking seriously about how to prepare physicians to function in this larger range of roles and these more complicated situations. Certainly, we will be continuing to prepare specialists of all kinds, but there is and will be a continuing role for generalists. It gets harder and harder to know what constitutes a good education for a generalist in our increasingly complicated times. Educating physicians to be able to survive and flourish in the midst of economic and financial conflicts is, I think, an important task for medical educators.

I have certain expectations for the future of medicine. There is no question that medical knowledge will continue to grow faster than the population and the economy. Technology, particularly computers, will accelerate the growth of medical knowledge. I think they will do more in that direction than they will in the direction of helping us to cope as individual human beings. The growth of medical knowledge and the development of new technologies will change the roles of physicians toward those qualities of human beings that current machines do not possess: breadth of perception, capacity to perform many different kinds of actions, physical actions, recognizing and accommodating to new situations, awareness of emotions, empathy, and encouragement.

By changing roles for physicians, this rise of technology will of necessity modify the goals of medical education. The education of physicians is becoming as much more complicated and difficult and challenging as the practice of medicine. It is on this that the medical schools and universities should be focusing, rather than on functioning primarily as regulators of physician supply.

I agree that we are entering a time of intense conflict within medicine, but I am also reminded that Martin Luther King once said that all confrontations ultimately lead to progress. This may be a difficult time for physicians and medical professionals but it is a great time for medicine. As Dr. Sammons put it, it has never been better and it is going to be better still. We stand at the threshold of medicine for the twenty-first century that is of a power and subtlety and an effectiveness that our forebears simply could not have imagined.

We in medicine will, of course, continue to live with the uncertainty and the unknown. Every sick human being is an utterly unique person bringing an utterly new situation to the doctor. Perhaps one sign of progress is that we are more conscious of our ignorance. What the future requires is intelligent, imaginative, creative, energetic, dedicated human beings. It is the job of the private medical schools to prepare such persons to practice in the future.

IV. From a Public Medical School

M. ROY SCHWARZ, M.D.

First, let us discuss the dimensions of the public medical education enterprise. There are seventy-five state-supported or public medical schools in this country. They train 60 percent (40,801) of the medical students; they employ 51 percent (28,835) of the faculty; and they educate 40 percent (28,744) of the house staff. The average budget of the state medical school is $59.2 million, of which $20 million (33 percent) comes from state sources.

There are forty-five private schools. They have 40 percent of the students, 49 percent of the faculty, and 33 percent of the residents, but they have an average budget of $72 million and on an average they get $2.2 million of state support.

In addition to those differences, there are three that you must know in order to understand the state medical educational system in this country. First, state medical schools have less management flexibility and less freedom than private schools; therefore, they do not respond to trends and changes as rapidly as private institutions.

The second difference is in the quality of leadership you can expect from the boards of trustees. Almost without exception, the boards that govern universities in the public sector are either political appointees or they are elected, often on partisan grounds. They often do not have the independent means, reputations, networks of contacts, and perspectives that are desired of board members. The decisions that they make are often made on partisan political grounds with little if any regard for educational merit or for national trends.

A third difference between public and private medical schools is that the state schools are exposed to public scrutiny in a way that private schools are not. Most state agencies, because of sunshine laws, cannot conduct any business in private.

What are the groups that can influence the decision of a public medical school if it is considering the possibility of altering its training capacity? First and foremost, there is the faculty which will, of course, ultimately make the decision. They vote on class size. The faculty are really led by administrators and, therefore, they are not independent organizations. Beyond that, there are some forces that are much greater than either of those two. There are the public officials: board members, governors, legislators, or members of the U.S. Congress.

Then there are the practicing physicians who can get at you through the legislature, the public, the referral of patients to private practitioners, and through their willingness or lack thereof to be involved in voluntary teaching. Add to that the alumni, the applicants and their families, community leaders and organizations, federal agencies through statutes, grants, programs, and regulations, and the donors.

Finally, there is the general public, who—through public officials, M.D.s, influential people, and, most important, the news media—can influence a decision that involves class size or the training capacity of the public medical schools.

What are the grounds on which people will make their decisions in this subject area? The first is their perception of health care needs. This may come as population/physician ratios, specialty and geographic distribution, care in the rural areas, changing demographics, technological changes, the roles of health professionals other than physicians, changes in the health care delivery system, corporatization of medicine, and behavior changes in physicians. An equally important reason, if not a more important one in the state system, is access. If you are insensitive to access you miss the game, because state universities are established to provide educational opportunities for the sons and daughters of the state.

For each entering physician in medical schools there are 14,000 people in this country. Therefore, if you are from a state like Colorado where the ratio is one to 23,000 or the state of Washington where it is one to 28,000, there is very little interest in decreasing class size, because it would be looked upon as further discriminating against state residents in terms of access, especially against those who do not have the financial means to apply and be competitive in the private market.

A third issue is economics. There is a growing opinion in the minds of many state legislators that reducing class size would save us some money in the medical schools. In fact, some have even gone so far as to suggest that we close the schools because we exist in an attractive area and we will have an influx of excess physicians from elsewhere without paying anything. How do you provide access under those conditions?

Another reason is that we have a tremendously good bargain for the care of the poor through our state-supported medical schools.

If the school of medicine did not provide this service through its faculty in their teaching hospital, we would have no equally viable economic option. Therefore, we must support the medical school. The most sophisticated economic view is that the very good state medical schools will take every dollar of state support that is given and they will multiply that four or five times with monies they get from elsewhere. Besides providing access to medical school for students, that investment will provide access to medical care for the poor and create jobs as well.

Those are the ostensible reasons for changing class size, but there are some even more important real reasons that nobody talks about and certainly nobody writes about. The first is the availability of physicians. This is characterized by Senator Magnuson who said to me, "Roy, as long as I have to wait two weeks to get an appointment and I have to wait two hours when I get there to see the doctor, we don't have enough!" If you add to that, "My doctor is too busy to explain to me what is going on and to listen to me," there is an availability perception that drives the need for more physicians.

The second real reason which is very rarely talked about is the image of physicians. If the image in a state is that doctors are insensitive and arrogant, that they are the primary cause of rising health care costs, and that they are more concerned about what they can get out of the system for their own welfare than what they can contribute to improve the welfare of their patients, then there is an automatic reaction to increase the number of physicians and drive down the amount of money that they make. That is a very real view that exists out there.

One thing that can override all of these economic factors is whether or not the important decision makers trust, respect, admire and, most importantly, like the leader of the medical school. If they do, they will accede to whatever that individual suggests.

What then can state medical schools do about managing this problem? First, if you wish to reduce class size for whatever reason, the best way to sell that idea is on economic grounds. First you must be certain that your small towns and inner cities are covered by manpower, that the physicians' image is manageable, and that the medical school leader is liked by the decision makers.

If you wish to maintain your class size, the best arguments are access to the sons and daughters of taxpayers and specialty and geographic maldistribution. A third argument is shifting trends. We are going to have more elderly, and the disease patterns are going to change as they need more health care. The fourth point is economic, the bargain basement opportunity for care of the poor.

If you wish to increase your class size, all I can recommend is that you pray. I can think of no good arguments for doing that at this time.

In summary, state medical schools are unique beasts. They occupy the majority of the medical education enterprise. They are driven in large part by the political winds, and many of the reasons that drive the politics are never clearly enunciated.

V. Third-Party Payment: Industry

WILLIS GOLDBECK

I think it would be a mistake for the folks in the medical, hospital, and educational worlds to seek a business voice on all of these complex issues. You are not going to find a single voice and that is just as well. You have to recognize that all business organizations do not have the same mission or philosophy. Their positions on a variety of health policy issues, of which these that we are discussing are just a couple, will not always appear to be totally consistent either with one another or with the medical community.

There are some common themes among the business community from which will probably emerge the majority of the public policy opinions on medical education and manpower. These include the attitudes that cost management is necessary, slow, complex, and expensive and will not go away and that cost management strategies can work, will work, and are going to be made to work.

Values and attitudes are changing within many of the elements of the business community. The attitude that the government is the enemy or is always bad is certainly no longer accepted, any more than the attitude that hospitals and doctors are ipso facto good is automatically accepted. The attitude that benefits are something to be given away and ignored has been replaced with the attitude that benefits are assets to be jointly managed with the employee.

More and more, businesses have the attitude that cost management can increase quality and should not be viewed as an automatic threat to quality. Many of these changes that are being brought about are increasing the quality of the care and the information about choices that patients, employees, and their families have. There is still a very large amount of waste that can be cut out of the system without hurting anybody.

We certainly do not know the number of physicians needed. We take rather small solace in the fact that neither economists nor physicians seem to know the number either. Space medicine and genetic engineering are two large question marks today that will be very prevalent forces in the next few years. It will be a terrible mistake to try to define a specific target number of any aspect of the medical profession.

We would agree with Dr. Sammons that there is not a defined amount of excess, nor do we think that there ought to be a single source that determines the amount of medical manpower in the United States in the coming decade. There is, however, evidence of a surplus already. If you work in the business community now and you are trying to start an HMO, doctors seek you out. Only a few years ago, those doctors felt that their employment and referral opportunities were being threatened by HMOs. It was a major political, economic, and professional fight to find somebody who would do the HMO job. Today, doctors come looking for the opportunity.

Corporate medical departments are now solicited by high quality young graduates of top medical schools in the country looking for work. Four or five years ago when we started instituting corporate wellness programs and went to some physicians seeking help, we were laughed out of the room; that was inappropriate for physicians. Today we get several calls every week from physicians asking if there is any company in America where they could get jobs as a wellness coordinator. So there is already very clear evidence of a surplus. There are also needs in the business community that are not being met, toxicology and mental health professionals being two glaring examples.

The business community tends to support continued funding for medical education and research. Those are areas the business community understands from the nature of its own work. That does not mean there is blind support for the status quo, either in terms of the teaching hospitals and medical educational institutions that exist today or for the idea that they have an automatic right to continue to exist.

There is a great deal of confusion about what constitutes appropriate or good medical education. We have no sense of what constitutes high-quality standards for medical education. We have heard consistently during this conference how 20 percent of the people coming out of school into the medical force are, by your own definitions, awful. They come from terrible schools outside the United States or from systems within the United States. We hear that they are not qualified, that they ought to be thrown out, that the licensing procedures should be changed. How are we supposed to know who to be served by and which educational institutions to support? When somebody suggests a 10 percent cutback, everybody rushes forward and says that is terrible because we have threatened medical education in America. Would it threaten it or would it help get rid of at least half of that terrible 20 percent? We do not know. If one wishes to build a political alliance with the business community on the future of medical education in America, someone had better come forth with what constitutes good medical education in America or anywhere else.

If you read the literature on medical education, you have to wonder whether or not medical education can possibly keep up with the information overload that physicians and other practitioners must face. Research shows that 40 percent of physicians acknowledge they cannot begin to keep up with their own profession. Ten thousand scientific journals are now being published which have some medical information in every issue. In addition, there are the computer influx and the telecommunications era.

A second critical area is the increasing demand for accountability from the profession. Ten years ago no business person in America could have told you anything about what his insurance purchased, other than how much it cost. Today, virtually any member of our group and lots of others can give you, by name, profiles of the physicians they pay for, what they do, how they do it, what they charge, and hospital profiles by DRG and by procedure, compared with every other medical group in America. Five years from now, individuals will be able to have on their home screen any profile of the activities of any element of the medical profession and algorithms of every aspect of self-care. The telecommunications revolution and the changing ownership of information will be among the greatest controlling factors of the future of medical education.

Many in the business community will favor regionalization of services and will not be overly concerned with the inability of a particular rural town to have the very latest of all aspects of the profession and the technology. The Metropolitan Opera is not in every town. No other aspect of our society is in every town, and all of medical care is not going to be in every town either.

One of the issues raised by the combination of concern about what constitutes good quality care and the accountability question is a growing wondering about standards of care. How does that relate to medical education? If the standard of care means that every town's community physicians are supposed to establish their own system of standards of quality, that must mean that there is no standard of what constitutes good education. We wonder sometimes why there is such a revulsion against the idea of more rational standards—not hard and fast rules to take the art away from medicine but at least the recognition that the science base is rather shaky. We see experiments that show that 50 percent of lab tests can be done away with, that it may be possible to do chemotherapy in half the time, that length of stay can be reduced by one-half or three-quarters or four-fifths in some cases; yet quality seems to go up in terms of outcomes. All of that was said to be impossible just a few years ago because it would be devastating for the patient, and yet it does not seem to be.

The inability to draw a clear connection between standards of care and how to reduce the malpractice problem is certainly something that all facets of the private sector will have to work on together.

I think you will see an increasing willingness within the corporate community to provide financial resources for real medical research rather than for buildings, bricks, and mortar.

Another factor that we must all consider is the growth of attention to prevention in the private sector and the business community. There is a much greater willingness on the part of many leaders in the business community to accept the contention that prevention deserves a higher degree of investment than it has had in the past. Of all of our medical complex in the United States, we still spend well less than 2 percent of our budget on prevention. In the standard industrial codes in the United States five years ago there was no code for anything to do with self-care, prevention, or fitness-oriented endeavors of business practices. Today, there is such a code and it is a more than $22 billion part of industry. This is a five-year growth not to be ignored. The fastest growing element is self-diagnostic medical equipment, equipment purchased by the individual, used without the presence of anybody who ever had a medical education or probably ever will have.

We in the business community have very clear evidence that

the medical profession will follow economic incentives. This is seen on the negative side when psychiatrists rush into Detroit as soon as there is a new benefit in the automotive industry insurance packet. This is seen on the positive side when a business changes its reimbursement package and finds that the doctors around its facilities are suddenly able to provide ambulatory surgery because it is now reimbursable. This is seen in the different responses of medical groups to apparently similar economic incentives. The mere fact that one hospital, faced with ambulatory surgicenter competitive pressures, feels it must raise its rates while another hospital with exactly the same circumstances feels it must lower its rates suggests that one cannot be automatically enamored with competition as the solution to everything but that solutions will be taken on a case-by-case basis.

You will find the business community increasingly involved in ethical issues and in those issues that business has allowed to be the purview of government: the area of uncompensated care or bad debt and charity care and the willingness to start to grapple with multitier methodologies in delivering care in the United States. We are going to be faced with the necessity of designing an acceptable lower level tier of care. It is a sham to pretend that we have one level of care in America when between 20 million and 35 million people do not have regular access to care. The mere fact that once in a great while they might get something good does not constitute an equal level of care. Designing well-managed care systems for those of lesser circumstances is a lot better than pretending that they have access to the same thing that everybody else has when that is simply not the case.

I think you are going to find business paying much more attention to the licensure issue. A typical reaction from businesses around the country is that they do not believe the licensure boards are very serious. We would certainly support toughening the licensing boards if they would then use that new backbone. By the same token, you will find a great deal of concern about any group that uses "acceptable character" as a methodology for shrinking or expanding access to the system.

You will find business increasingly involved in decisions about transplantation and other issues which previously had been considered to be government's decisions. Business involvement in issues like teenage pregnancy is going to become more and more prevalent. We find now in a number of companies that more than

25 percent of the births that they pay for are births to children of their employees, in effect for grandchildren.

I would urge you to remember the comments of Dr. Nicholson and others who have talked about the changing nature of values of work in America. It is probably useful to keep in mind that the white male is the minority worker in America today and that women are not going to be a legitimate excuse for the changing nature of medical education; rather they are the ones who will be in charge because of their greater numbers.

With the increases in longevity in the United States, I wonder if we are going to end up with the medical profession being one where age is aligned against participation or are we going to find out how to find useful activities within the healing arts for people in their sixties and their seventies and functional people in their eighties? Right now we have 40,000 people in America past the age of 100. By the end of this century, there will be over 100,000, and they are not all incapable.

By and large, business supports the development of nonphysician and limited-license providers as competitors. Business will not take the side of physicians in trying to stop the presence and growth of these practitioners.

You will find very little sympathy among the business community for the student debt issue. A $100,000 debt is actually no more than the typical small businessman in the United States has to incur, yet he has a fraction of the resources that will be present for every medical student who does reasonably well. On the other hand, this presents an opportunity, either by making the interest tax deductible or by forgiving the loan entirely, of having these doctors work outside of the United States in important areas of the world that need help. There are many ways the pressure of the loan can be turned into a positive step.

Few people in the business community are concerned about a reduction in the individual choice of patients as long as the choices that remain are better-informed choices. With the kinds of utilization and comparative data systems that are now available, we will be much better off giving somebody half a dozen choices of excellence than letting them wander through a maze of ignorance.

I think you will find that the major employers in America do not pay much attention to insurance carriers anymore. They are not the deciding voice they used to be. By and large the big corporations are going to make their own decisions and hire or not hire carriers who will do their bidding rather than the other way around.

I think you will not find the business community thinking that physician surpluses should be a cause of fear. If physicians are working fewer hours, that would generally be viewed as positive, because there will be more attention paid to individuals and more opportunities for physicians to pay attention to the other factors of life that could make them better-rounded individuals.

VI. Law

CLARK C. HAVIGHURST, J.D.

I had expected my role to be that of a wet blanket, dampening a general enthusiasm for private sector efforts to solve this problem of a physician excess. Yet hearing from the major professional organizations at this meeting, I do not sense any great desire to try to solve this problem by any action that would raise serious problems under the antitrust laws. The lack of propensity to pursue some of the strategies that I will be discussing may be attributable to the good legal advice these organizations receive, but I also do not sense any great frustration about the law and what it seems to require, although the FTC has been mentioned a few times in a critical way.

Let me suggest some hypothetical actions that the industry might take and discuss their legal status. The first idea might be to have the medical schools agree to cut back on enrollment. It would be very difficult to get the public medical schools to agree to this strategy, and they train the majority of students. Nevertheless, if the medical schools did attempt to solve the problem by such collective action, their agreement would be an agreement among competitors to reduce output and would probably be illegal. According to the Supreme Court, Congress, in the Sherman Act, has chosen competition as the way to run the economy and allows competition to engage in collective action only if it leaves the market free to function. If it impairs the functioning of the market, it is illegal, and they cannot argue that you did it for a worthy purpose. Thus, any claim that unrestricted competition among the medical schools for students is not in the public interest must be directed to Congress and cannot be made to the courts.

Medical schools could argue that they are not really engaged in a commercial enterprise and therefore are not required by the antitrust laws to compete. A few lower courts have suggested as much, as in the case of *Selman v. Harvard Medical School*. The plaintiff, Selman, was a USFMG studying at Guadalajara. He complained that he had been boycotted by the major medical schools when he sought to transfer back to a U.S. school at the end of his second year. The alleged boycott occurred at the time when Congress had offered subsidies to schools to expand their third-year classes in the hope that they would bring these USFMGs home and give them at least two years of quality education. The leading medical schools boycotted that program, however, deciding collectively that they would not allow themselves to be bribed to bend their admission standards by Congress's subsidies.

Selman lost his case when the court said that the admissions criteria that were the subject of dispute were "a non-commercial aspect of the practice of the learned profession" and that the boycott had "a purely incidental effect on the commercial aspects of the medical profession." I do not think this rationale would apply to an effort by medical schools to limit the number of physicians turned out. Such an agreement would have a direct, not an incidental, effect on "the commercial aspects of the medical profession."

I also think that, although the court in the *Selman* case reached the right result, it did so for the wrong reason. For one thing, the court focused its attention on the boycott's effects on consumers of medical care but ignored the effects on consumers of medical education—people like Selman himself. One might have thought that Selman and others like him were entitled, in a competitive world, to have the benefit of independent decisions by medical schools on their qualifications. You must assume, I think, that the courts will eventually recognize education as a commercial activity or at least an activity in which competition can be unlawfully impaired. To the extent that the *Selman* court held otherwise, it may have gotten it wrong. There is another ground, however, for the result reached.

The antitrust laws have long been construed not to apply to collective action to achieve some political objective. Although it is debatable whether a boycott (as opposed to other kinds of concerted action) can be justified on the ground that the partner was only trying to achieve a political result, it seems to me that the medical schools in the *Selman* case were engaged in a political protest and should be protected on this account. The point is simply that the Sherman Act, which deals with market behavior, should not be construed to apply to collective action of a political kind.

This principle turns out to be quite important in evaluating the things the industry might do collectively to deal with the doctor glut. Because competitors can act together in good faith to seek legislative or other public action on any problem—even if the action turns out to benefit them at the expense of their competitors —there is a rather broad area of activity that they can engage in under the antitrust laws without serious problems. The only caveat is that they must avoid falling under what is called the "sham exception." That means that they must really be seeking a political result, not conspiring to eliminate competition directly.

Another way in which the industry might try to curb oversupply is through its control over specialty training. The number of residencies could be limited by accrediting fewer programs or by persuading the existing programs to reduce the number of positions. I think it would be very difficult to defend a denial of accreditation to a school if there was any basis for suspecting that it reflected a desire to limit the number of physicians turned out. If training programs are turned down or told to reduce their size, you would need good reasons related to the quality of training in order to avoid losing an antitrust case and you would probably get sued in any event. As hospitals begin to feel competitively disadvantaged they will be more inclined to bring such a case, and the problems could be very great. Those cases are costly to defend even if you win, and your motives would be very closely scrutinized.

In writing about accrediting recently, I argued that lawfully constituted private bodies ought to be rather free to express their views on training programs by means of accreditation or the denial thereof and that accrediting ought not to be closely regulated by courts. That has not been generally accepted as a principle, however, and I do not think you can count on it.

Another strategy for controlling the numbers of physicians might be for a specialty board to try to increase the difficulty or the cost of entering the specialty by extending the period of training. This method would include the practice of "grandfathering," that is, increasing the requirements for new entrants without providing for recertifying those who are already in the specialty. Raising training requirements to reflect increasing complexity in a particular discipline is one thing; doing it to keep down the number of competitors is another. If there was any evidence that concern over the doctor glut inspired a change in accreditation or certification requirements, that would expose you to serious risk. If you think about it, it would be pretty scary to face a class action brought on behalf of an entire class or several classes of residents who had been required to undergo an extra year of training. If they should win by showing that you had an anticompetitive purpose, they would be entitled to recover three times their lost earnings during that extra year of training plus their legal fees. If you add up that amount for a whole class of residents in a large specialty, it is a frightening amount.

One other way in which the physician glut could be addressed locally is through withholding hospital staff privileges. Although a medical staff is not free to close itself, it could perhaps persuade the governing board of the hospital to close the staff or put a moratorium on adding doctors to the staff, at least in certain specialties. The hospital would have to be motivated by its own interest, not by the doctors' interest, and it would have to show that quality and efficiency were enhanced by that move. But, like an HMO, a hospital ought to be free to select the staff it needs to take care of the patients it has. I think that hospitals do have that kind of freedom. The principle that private institutions and health plans and others are free to select providers and to turn down those they do not need is really the market's way of promoting efficiency and tailoring supply to demand in a local market. Although the antitrust laws have occasionally been invoked by those trying to get into a market, it seems to me a spurious use of antitrust law, and I think we are coming to a better understanding that would-be entrants can be turned away for business reasons without antitrust consequences.

VII. State Government

EUGENE S. MAYER, M.D.

My first point is that if states are to play a responsible role in medical education, it will be in those states in which a partnership of forces—including the academic health science centers, organized medicine, hospitals, and perhaps even the business community and others—can speak with a reasonably common voice that we will see the development of responsible steps with funding, which will help moderate the number of students and rearrange the specialty mix if that is what that particular state needs.

My second point is that despite our moving into an era of limited resources, we have not fully left the era of social justice described by Dr. Anlyan. This means that our partnership of forces will have to show state legislatures that we will not backslide in relation to progress underway and systems in place but will continue to improve social justice as we move to effect new strategies.

The basis for my observations concerning the role of states and the importance of partnerships in moving our state legislatures comes from fifteen years of creating, nurturing, and expanding partnerships in North Carolina, which have helped reach collective agreement on strategies resulting in substantial continuing state funding to all our institutions. These partnerships also concern themselves with the supply of physicians, address the issue of geographic and specialty distribution, and work to improve the quality of medical education and care in the state.

Decisions to alter the patterns of medical education and residency training at the state level will not be easy for at least three reasons. First, some states are still trying to meet their manpower goals of the seventies. Second, some states are aware that there is a national component to the problem and they will want to see momentum on a national basis before they make major changes. Third, and perhaps more important, state legislatures will have difficulty understanding the issue and interpreting the data.

In Figure 19 are two lines and a period of time that goes from 1970 to 1980 on the bottom. The top line looks at the physician/population ratio in the sixty most rural counties in North Carolina. We are the fourth most rural state. The bottom line is an average for 760 comparable rural counties of the United States. These data show our legislators substantial progress in the improvement of the physician/population ratio in our most rural counties, one of the things they wanted us to accomplish. While I believe that this is consistent with Professor Newhouse's market theory, there is also a series of program strategies that have helped bring this about in addition to market forces.

If we go one step further with our data and look at figure 20, we can see how much the physician/population ratios have improved statewide by comparing 1963–73 with 1973–83. Even in this very rural state the improvement in the physician/population ratio in our rural counties is, in fact, a statewide phenomenon. These are good signs to legislators and to those of us who have been working to bring this about.

There were essentially six strategies that our state government collectively agreed to that helped to bring about these accomplishments in addition to whatever benefits we gained from market forces and from being in the Sunbelt. There were the rural health strategy focusing on primary care center development and physician recruitment; physician extender support strategy; family medicine and primary care training strategies; dollars to build a new medical school and to support expansion of all three existing schools, with a special emphasis on North Carolina residents; a clear minority recruitment strategy for medical schools; and a statewide area health education center program that in many ways helps to bring many of the previous strategies together.

The Area Health Education Center (AHEC) program is designed to bring the educational process closer to the practicing physician and health professionals in all 100 counties in the state. By linking the four academic health centers to all towns of the state through nine regional education training centers—which look like mini-academic health science centers with facilities, faculty, and libraries, and the $24 million continuing state appropriation—we are able to expose academia to the community and the

Figure 19. Physician/10,000 Population Ratio for Nonmetropolitan Counties in North Carolina and the United States, 1970–80. North Carolina nonmetropolitan counties have shown continued improvement in their average physician/population ratios while comparable nonmetropolitan counties in the rest of the United States have shown only slight improvement in their average ratios.

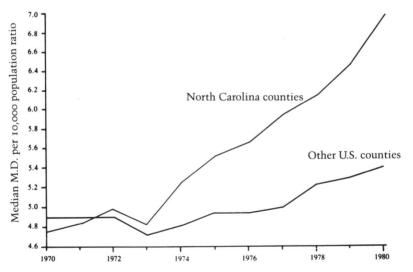

Figure 20. Change in Physician/Population Ratio by County, 1963–83.

During 1963–73, before the development of the statewide AHEC Program, 43 counties experienced a worsening physician-to-population ratio; the ratio for 16 counties was unchanged and 41 counties experienced an improved ratio.

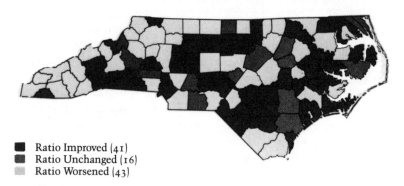

■ Ratio Improved (41)
▩ Ratio Unchanged (16)
▨ Ratio Worsened (43)

Change in Physician/Population Ratio by County, 1973–83.

During the period 1973–83, after the creation of the statewide AHEC Program, the Office of Rural Health Services, and other health manpower programs, 89 counties experienced an improved physician-to-population ratio, the ratio for 4 counties was unchanged, and the ratio worsened in only 7 counties.

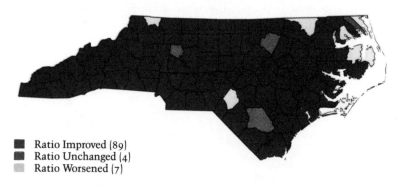

■ Ratio Improved (89)
▩ Ratio Unchanged (4)
▨ Ratio Worsened (7)

Total active nonfederal physicians
Sources: American Medical Association; Health Services Center, UNC-Chapel Hill.

community to academia on a daily basis (figure 21). This strategy also includes a $4.5 million component to support statewide primary care residency development, and we have made considerable progress toward some of the goals that Dr. Petersdorf put before us with respect to primary care/specialty balance.

There are sixteen other states that currently have about $18 million of federal AHEC money and, in addition, find their states and localities supporting the program to the tune of another $150 million, which I believe is a testimony to Congressman Rogers and his committees that helped create this program.

In the aggregate, our state legislature has increased the supply of physicians and other health professionals. It has reordered primary care specialty training so that we have a position in primary care for more than 50 percent of our statewide graduates from all four medical schools. It has created a network of regional education and training centers with support services which help attract and retain young physicians and help decrease their professional isolation. It has seen a significant increase in the retention of medical students from all of our schools and of residents in training throughout the state; this is particularly notable in towns of fewer than five thousand people.

There are many counties in North Carolina that still have population/primary care physician ratios of greater than 2,500 to one. While figure 19 showed tremendous progress, and we take

Figure 21. Counties Served by the North Carolina Area
Health Education Centers Program.

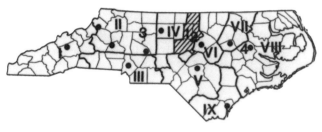

I. Mountain AHEC
II. Northwest AHEC
III. Charlotte AHEC
IV. Greensboro AHEC
V. Fayetteville AHEC
VI. Wake AHEC
VII. Area L AHEC
VIII. Eastern AHEC
IX. Wilmington AHEC

Location of university medical centers: (1) U.N.C. at Chapel Hill, (2) Duke, (3) Bowman Gray, (4) East Carolina University.

pride in that, remember that that is the trend line. There is still a lot of unfinished business and figure 20 is a representation of that. If you were a state legislator in North Carolina, would you want to decrease our class size? As always, the choices for our legislators are difficult ones. If we have difficulty agreeing on the solutions and even, in fact, agreeing on the problems, imagine how our legislators will feel when confronted with data showing both sufficiency of supply and continuing shortages.

If we hope to convince state legislators to make shifts in their policies, we need to be armed with several sets of evidence. First, we need to speak to progress made relative to the 1970 manpower goals that we once developed with our legislators. Second, we must show the potential for physician/population ratios to go beyond reasonable limits in a majority of the state's communities, not in a few. We should couple these data with other data to show the potential negative impact of these ratios on both cost and quality. Third, we must show that the major professional associations, the academic health science centers, and the hospitals are speaking with one voice. We have done that in this state for a decade, and I believe that we need to keep it going. I think this would be true for other states as well. We also need to show that some efforts are under way to effect a national solution to some of these problems. Fourth, we must give evidence to our general assemblies that we have mechanisms to continue to assess areas of unmet needs and that we have mechanisms, through our programs, to address these needs. Finally, we must show that whatever we do to change numbers, we are still affording reasonable access for sons and daughters of legislators and others to have an opportunity to pursue a medical education.

Sophisticated state legislators will want to see that their earlier efforts to improve supply, distribution, and quality will continue through activities that enhance the retention of physicians who have now begun to settle in some of our underserved areas; activities that will continue to augment the quality of their practice; and activities that will keep the academic center in the community setting without retreating to the ivory tower. In other words, changes in manpower strategy will need to recognize, build upon, and maintain structures that have been put into place to meet 1970 goals while shaping these structures to meet the demographic and manpower challenges of the nineties.

The importance of our state legislatures is clear. Our success in working with them to change manpower policies will depend on our data, our seriousness of purpose in the public interest, and our degree of partnership in speaking with one voice. Partnerships were relatively easy to effect in an era of expanding resources, yet even so, academic health science centers, professional associations, and hospitals in some states never achieved these partnerships. In our state, we are proud that we did.

Can such partnerships be created and/or sustained now in an era of limited resources? For the sake of the academic health science center, the medical profession, and the care of our patients, we have no choice but to assure their continued development or our disparate voices will hardly rally state legislators to progressive manpower strategies.

Discussion

DR. DAVID J. OTTENSMEYER: Our discussion has been about the possible surplus of physicians and, in my view, we are just about where we were at the beginning when Dr. Anlyan said that it had to do with what the policy of the country is as far as funding health care is concerned. If the present policy of funding and reimbursement persists, the evidence suggests that there will be a surplus of physicians in this country. Out in the communities we already see a plateau in the income of physicians. Some physicians have had a 10 to 15 percent absolute decrease of income in the past three years. As a result of shifts of market share or the introduction of HMOS, some physicians have lost 30 percent of their practice in a period of only weeks. I expect to see data that will show declines in the absolute income of physicians of 3 to 5 percent per year. The importance of our discussion is how the profession is going to respond to that.

I can particularly relate to some of the things that Dr. Tosteson said about the impact of corporate medical care in our society, especially in our urban areas, and the question of how our allies in the medical education business are going to respond to it. The health care organizations, including those controlled, managed, and led by physicians, are making logical and informed decisions in their own self-interest about how their future will be ordered financially and organizationally. That can only hasten and facilitate this whole process that has been called corporate medical practice. The medical profession now must ask itself what it is going to do, how it is going to influence and mold that process. The development and evolution of corporate entities entering into health care is extremely important to us.

We must not ignore our potential role in this development. We should not ignore our tradition and history and such value-laden beliefs as commitments to the voluntary system or the fee-for-service system or individual choice. These things are too important for the medical profession to leave to the lawyers, hospitals, hospital administrators, and MBAS.

One of the things that medical schools could be looking at is how they can prepare physicians to have a role in the development of health care organizations. We have traditionally considered the role of the physician to be that of a clinician, yet the American Medical Association has gradually acknowledged that there are other important constituencies in medicine. They have brought into their umbrella organization nonscientific constituencies, such as the women's medical association, the physician lawyers, the American Academy of Medical Directors, and the American Group Practice Association. These are the people who are taking on a leadership and management role in the development of these new corporations; that is an important role that the profession needs to think about now. Eventually there may well be a specialty of medical management. If nothing else, as the surplus develops we may be able to use some of the surplus physicians as administrators.

DR. RICHARD G. WILBUR: Almost our entire discussion has been concerned with the intake of medical students—how many are coming in—and very little discussion has concerned what should happen to all those who are already in the entire pool of physicians—soon to be 600,000. We have a partial consensus that the only active way in which we can limit intake would be on the basis of quality. But the marketplace, competition, and conflict will not only limit intake; it will also affect those who are already in the pool. So why should quality concerns not affect those of us already in practice? Why are we exempt?

Historically there is a reason: we are a learned profession; we are taught over a period of time; we are examined and measured; and it is made certain that we have been taught well for a progressively longer period of time. Then we are set free on society with relatively few limitations, unless we do something quite bad or unless we wish to do something rather complex within a well-run hospital. Dr. Galusha and the Federation of State Medical Boards are doing their best but are seriously limited by laws and lawyers. Dr. Hanlon referred to the American College of Surgeons' efforts, which are also hampered by laws and lawyers. Dr. Sammons spoke to the need for equal qualifications among foreign medical graduates and LCME graduates.

I am suggesting that we need equity between the young and the old, between those coming in and those of us who are already in. One of the major problems, of course, is assessing quality. The present systems assessing quality are more systems of measuring whether one has acquired information and some ability to manipulate it within the medical school and residency training than they are related to the actual practice of medicine. A recent American Board of Pediatrics examination had one-third of its questions regarding a certain genetic defect that is encountered in about three-tenths of 1 percent of the patients coming to see the average physician. That examination hardly determines whether or not a practicing pediatrician is doing a good job with his patients.

People like Dr. Satcher and others have made great efforts to bring into medicine physicians who will work in underserved areas and take special care of those people. It would be wrong to put these doctors out of practice because of their failure to show intellectual brilliance in answering questions irrevelant to their daily practice in medicine. I am not suggesting that intellectual brilliance is antithetical to good practice performance, but much of the time it certainly is not directly necessary; other qualities are probably more valuable.

One thing that we can do is to set up better standards of physician performance for everyone—young or old, foreign or U.S. medical graduate, male or female, majority or minority—by which we should all be measured. This may well reduce the number of physicians. Whether or not it does, it certainly will increase the quality of care, which is what the medical schools and residency training programs should be trying to attain in the end anyway.

MR. C. DOUGLAS EAVENSON: The surplus of physicians, if there is one, will certainly be a concern of business and industry if it results in increased costs without an increase in quality. But the surplus could result in competition because of the increased numbers, and that increased competition could be good. The point has been made that HMOS, PPOS, and other entities of that sort find it much easier to get good qualified providers today than in times past.

Our discussions have focused on making it more difficult to get into the system. I think Dr. Wilbur's suggestion is one that I would also raise: Why not make it more difficult to stay in or easier to get rid of those who give medicine a bad name? Why not use this surplus as a basis for trying to get rid of the "bad guys"? There are certainly examples of physicians who deal in inappropriate services and numbers of tests, and surgeries by podiatrists who do a toe at a time; Caesarean sections with hysterectomies and D&CS. When you look at those procedures and the patterns of practice in various parts of the country, you have to wonder why they vary so much. You usually find the cause to be the economic incentive.

We also have the problem of doctors who casually sign sick slips for leave; maybe that is not per se a part of health care costs but it certainly has an impact on the cost of doing business. The folks who get primarily exercised about some of these things are those who are picking up the bills—the business men and the insurance carriers—but we do not see much activity on the part of the medical community in trying to police its own ranks.

DR. DAVID SATCHER: In asking the question, What are the important issues to confront regarding the physician supply? it seems as if there are three issues that we can talk about: cost, quality, and equity. The issue of cost has been discussed extensively. We have also had some discussion on quality; we would all tend to agree that the issue of quality is a very complicated one and that our approach to it is not always objective. Even though we try to be objective, we are influenced by our background. I think quality is critical and always has to be kept in the forefront.

The issue of equity is interesting to me because I came into medicine at a time when that issue was at the forefront. I remember in 1968 when the National Medical Association (NMA), the AMA, and the AAMC, along with the federal government and foundations, agreed on some very clear goals having to do with equity of access to medical education and to medical care. It might be the only time that those organizations have agreed on anything so extensively. There was a lot of idealism and enthusiasm at that time, and I think we have lost a lot of that in medicine today.

I think the issue of equity is not a dead issue in this country. Secretary Heckler, in her report to Congress last year, pointed out that there is a persistent gap in health status in this country between whites and nonwhites. She especially pointed to the differential in life expectancy, infant mortality, and prevalence of diseases. Infant mortality, for example, is still twice as great among blacks in this country as among others. The life expectancy of the black man in some of the rural communities of the South, especially in places like Georgia and Tennessee, is, in fact, worse than it is in Kenya. There are some striking issues having to do with equity of access to care that cannot be completely separated from issues having to do with equity of access to health professional education. As they were in 1968, they are clearly related today. It is important that medical education and the medical profession not become elite in terms of this issue of access; I think there is a danger of that happening if we are not careful. I still believe that the National Health Service Corps was a good idea and even though it did not work the way we wanted it to, I believe that we should have made some changes to make it work.

Perhaps an international health service corps is an idea whose time has come. We have talked a lot about foreign medical graduates and the fact that so many of them come from countries where they *are* needed to this country where they are *not* needed. Perhaps it is time for us to look at the possibility of sending people the other way. One way to do that would be with an international health service corps that deals with problems not only in West Africa and East Africa and other places, but also in underserved communities in this country. We could reward and provide incentives for people to deal with these underserved communities.

I hope that, as we deal with this question of How many physicians do we need? and the growing number of physicians, we will keep in mind all three of these issues: cost, quality, and equity.

MS. RITA WROBLEWSKI: It is not clear that we all agree what the problem is. For example, Mr. Havighurst talked about the doctor glut, and yet there has been no unanimity of opinion that there is a doctor glut, just that the supply of physicians in the United States is increasing.

Now we are talking about opportunities and that fits in with how we plan a business. First, we talk about the problems and then we talk about the opportunities. In fact, Mr. Goldbeck talked about student loans not necessarily being a problem but an issue that could be turned into an opportunity.

I suppose our disquiet is understandable because we are going through a period of rapid change, and change always makes people uncomfortable, particularly people who have a lot to lose by potential change. There is an assumption, I think, that the physician belongs in a particular role in the social structure, deserving high income and status. Perhaps it behooves us to question that very specifically. Underlying some of the disquiet was perhaps the concern that the physician would lose some of that very special status that he has had in the past.

Dr. Tosteson talked about conflict leading to progress. I think

Dickens said it better than all of us: "It was the best of times, it was the worst of times." There are some special opportunities for those of us working in many sectors, and I think it is important that we do work together. Dr. Mayer talked about the partnership of forces. If we all go away thinking that the many sectors represented here have worked together on issues of mutual interest to make for progress, I think we will have accomplished a great deal.

Dr. Tosteson also talked about corporate medicine. Rather than railing against it, we might try to maximize whatever is positive in the development of corporate medicine and minimize the negative developments. Corporate medicine would like to work with academic medicine, and there must be issues of mutual interest that they can work on together. That is also true of industry in general, working together toward the support of research. Perhaps corporate medicine can get more involved in the care of the poor and the underserved and be integrated into the health care system in a wholesome way.

PROFESSOR ROSEMARY A. STEVENS: Conclusion number one that I hear is that medical care decisions are really financial decisions, period. The second conclusion is that we really do not know how many physicians we need. The third conclusion is that the traditional mechanisms for deciding how many physicians we need through the professional associations are illegal. Fourth, all this could lead to bafflement and inertia among the organizations that have traditionally been concerned with questions of physician supply and distribution.

I have also heard four very interesting calls for some sort of action on policy. The first is the need for outcomes research as to what are the effects of different forms of practice and what is the perceived quality of care under different conditions.

The second conclusion that I have heard in terms of action is the need for a major reappraisal of the structure and quality of specialists' education in residency training programs. Dr. Wilbur mentioned one aspect of that in terms of the relationship between the quality of education and testing and the quality of practice. It may very well be time for a major reappraisal across the board for specialist education programs.

The third clear policy we have agreed on is a much better articulation of policy toward USFMGs and the nature, standards, conditions, and effects of the offshore schools.

The fourth is the need for an international policy for medical education which is clearly related to decisions that are going to be made about physician production and distribution in the United States. This is not only a policy for the training of foreigners in the United States—which I worry we are going to neglect because of a backlash against foreign medical graduates—but also an international policy toward medical education that, as Dr. Satcher said, could work both ways.

DR. ARNOLD S. RELMAN: I would like to ask Professor Havighurst whether he heard anything illegal in Dr. Petersdorf's proposal. If the U.S. Congress, in modifying Medicare payments, set up a mechanism that said "We will only pay for house staff services in teaching hospitals under certain conditions," and if those conditions were to resemble in principle the conditions that Dr. Petersdorf described, would that be struck down by the courts?

PROFESSOR CLARK C. HAVIGHURST: There is no problem as far as I can see. It is always open to Congress to write a statute that is not consistent with the Sherman Act, and if one then construes the Sherman Act as having been amended or repealed for that kind of activity, there is no problem. There might be other legal challenges to the legislation, but there would be no violation of antitrust law if it were done correctly.

DR. ARNOLD S. RELMAN: So, the warning that you gave us—that attempts by the private sector to regulate numbers of physicians would be illegal—simply reflects a prior decision made by the U.S. Congress, and the problem then might be resolved, conceivably, by the U.S. Congress if it wished to. Is that correct?

PROFESSOR CLARK C. HAVIGHURST: Yes. I was speaking only about initiatives that the private sector might take without legislative authorization.

PROFESSOR ELI GINZBERG: We started with the question, Is there a surplus? and we came to no agreement. Then we were told that the supply is going up but we really do not know what the consequences of that are, so we walked away from that. Then we asked whether we want to do anything about the supply going up and we have said probably not. Then we came to the conclusion that we might not be able to do anything about the consequences of the supply going up even if we wanted to.

We all agreed that the FMG problem was an important one, but when we came to look at it more closely there was a great degree of unease about how we would grapple with it and whether we could get agreements about grappling with it, especially now when most of the FMGS are USFMG problems. Then Professor Havighurst warned us we cannot do anything very easily in the private sector market without getting into trouble with the law.

Then we all said we wanted to do something about quality, but nobody really knows what quality is, so we are not going to do much about quality.

My answers are, therefore, as follows. The reason we have been in such difficulties intellectually are, first, that the surplus question hinges on the continuance of money flowing into the system. If the money flows continue rapidly we will never have a surplus or we will never recognize it. Those declines in income that we have talked about will not occur in any significant fashion.

The second point is that we do not really know how much the market is being restructured in terms of so-called managed care. We have had absolutely wild notions put before us that half of the country will be in HMOs relatively quickly. I do not believe a word of it. If we knew what the money flow was and if we understood how far the restructuring problem is going to move and in what fashion, then, and only then, would there be a precondition to make adjustments on manpower supply. Then we could go to the state legislatures or back to the Congress and say this, that, or the other thing ought to happen. But, in the absence of any clarity with respect to money flows and restructuring, we cannot grapple with the manpower issue forthrightly and directly.

DR. BRYANT L. GALUSHA: Let me make the generic statement that medical licensing boards have been much more active in recent years. In 1982 there were 861 disciplinary actions nationwide reported to my office; in 1983 there were 1,041; and in 1984 there were 1,426. Some of this is due to better reporting, but clearly some of it is due to the increased activity of boards.

Medical licensing and disciplinary boards, in trying to perform their responsibilities expeditiously for the public, are hobbled by three main things. The first is financial constraints. The finances for boards come from physicians in registration fees. Unfortunately, a lot of these are sequestered by state government and used for other things. The second is the Medical Practice Act. A board can be no better than the authority vested in its Medical Practice Act.

Third is our current legal system. One of the last cases I sat on in North Carolina went up to the Supreme Court and took six years. I just sat in on a case in Texas, where one of the attorneys said to the board after five days of keeping five laymen and five physicians away from their practices, "I'm going to wear you out until you compromise!"

Let me assure you that medical licensing boards are aware of the problem and they are becoming more active.

DR. JAMES H. SAMMONS: There is a gleam out there someplace and the gleam is the Health Policy Agenda for the American People, which is two years under way with almost a year to go. It involves the United States government; AAMC, AHA, AMA, and every specialty organization in medicine, nursing, etc.; industry, the business roundtable, the U.S. Chamber of Commerce; and a wide variety of other people. Part of its activity is addressing the questions of health manpower and health education and its financing.

Although some people may be discouraged that we arrived at no fast and ready answers during this conference, the discussion is not over—it goes on. The Health Policy Agenda activity is a very rigorous activity and all of the participants, including the government representatives, are very vigorous participants.

MR. JACK K. SHELTON: It is true that the rate of increase in health care costs has flattened out. But there is another problem on the horizon that is going to cause the health care cost issue to become a very serious concern to the businessman: the accounting standards are being changed and there soon will be a requirement that businesses begin to at least look for a fund for the health care cost of their retirees. We have not precisely priced that out at Ford Motor Company but, as of right now, it looks like something over $4 billion. When these numbers begin to hit the balance sheets there is going to be increasing concern and worry about health care costs and, needless to say, increased action.

The market place is beginning to deal with this problem of manpower through limited-access plans. These are full-service limited-access plans like HMOs and PPOs, and there are also special benefit-capitated programs like lab services, dental, drugs, and so forth. The development of these programs is being enhanced and facilitated by the fact that employers, like Ford Motor Company, have on-line capability to run profiles on every provider of services to our employees. We are able to identify providers we think are cost efficient. Working with consultants from the medical community, we are going to be able to develop our own limited-access plans and fine tune those plans as data permit. As more and more limited-access plans come along and HMO growth continues, what is left in the fee-for-service area is going to be the least efficient part of the system. That means there is going to be substantial cost shifting to the traditional fee-for-service.

I would like to challenge my provider community friends to work with us in the business community to make sure we do not do the wrong things because we do not always know the right answers. We are going to move. We have to move. Our costs have reached a point where we must respond. Our Japanese counterparts have health care costs six times lower than ours. We have a very serious cost problem with our Japanese competitors, and health care is one piece of it.

I would urge you representatives of various organizations to find a businessman and work with him so that he will not do the wrong thing; he *is* going to do something.

DR. ROBERT G. PETERSDORF: First, none of you has convinced me that there is no doctor surplus. Those of us in the field who are training physicians and who are seeing them come out find Dr. Sammons to be out of tune with his major constituents, the medical associations. The California Medical Association, which did a very careful survey, said quite unequivocally in its manpower report that there are too many doctors in California, particularly too many surgeons.

My second point concerns Dr. Satcher's comment about international medicine. Having our young physicians serve overseas would be one way, at least for a finite period of time, to decompress the system. The Swiss, for instance, are thinking about doing it. If a significant number of our graduating seniors were to give three years of service overseas at a very modest stipend, they would do the world a lot of good and they would make a lot of sick people better.

But what do they do when they come back? In this uncertain time, the jobs are going to be harder to find, I cannot advise my son, who is finishing his residency training, to go to Africa for three years, because I have no idea what kind of job he will get when he comes back. That is one problem that our young people are facing: the uncertainty. The turmoil is affecting their natural desire to do good things.

Finally, I think the only thing that depressed me about this conference was the conclusion of our legal counsel. I guess he told us that in the private sector, within which most of us practice and work, the only route we can take to effect any major change is by government regulation and legislation. Otherwise we will be sued. That depresses me acutely.

DR. RICHARD H. EGDAHL: First, I don't know whether Professor Ginzberg or Dr. Ellwood is right about the growth of HMOs. Since I believe fee-for-service still has a lot of vitality, I would predict that we will see the major growth in a fee-for-service, well organized sector with management structures that will rise to meet the real need of personalized contact with physicians, because humane care by an individual is still very important. Unstructured fee-for-service is simply not competitive with multispecialty group practice but it can be made so by an appropriate organizational mode.

Second, I think we have grossly underestimated the power of the nonphysician health care professional—the nurses, social workers, and psychologists. The issues of comparable worth are floating throughout all industry, including the medical profession. We must come to grips with the fact that much of the care that we have traditionally given will be taken over, or is very much sought after by a group, largely of women, in some of the other health professions.

And, finally, if we are going to get an accurate fix on the numbers of doctors needed, keeping in mind what Dr. Nicholson has said about life-styles among younger physicians, we must also consider the physicians who are preparing for a second simultaneous career. Unless we know how many physicians will be involved part-time in some other service industry, we will be grossly overestimating the number of doctors needed.

DR. DANIEL C. TOSTESON: It seems to me that Dr. Petersdorf's proposal of three years of residency for all LCME graduates is not a manpower-regulating tool but an educational strategy. Underlying the proposal is the idea that all physicians, no matter what specialty they might enter, should prepare to be able to deliver a certain level of primary care or general practice. That is a very important strategic issue which deserves serious consideration in its own right, independent of the question of regulating the numbers of future physicians. On the financing side, to accept the notion that the federal government will be a money source and not a regulator is, to put it mildly, to fly in the face of experience!

Both Mr. Goldbeck and Mr. Whitehead gave us the image of computer-assisted self-care software programs that will provide patients with information that will enable them to do a lot for themselves that they are not able to do now. This is one example of the phenomenon of living in a knowledge age. The knowledge business is no longer going to be monopolized by institutions that specialize in knowledge. The profession, certainly the educational institutions, should embrace that, encourage it, and build on it. We will always need experts and those who are truly sophisticated in the field. We should strongly support that kind of development because it will improve the health of the people.

PROFESSOR ALAIN C. ENTHOVEN: Mr. Shelton just dropped a huge bombshell, and I do not know if many people noticed it. He said that the present value of the liability of the Ford Motor Company to pay for the future medical care of its retirees, net of what Medicare will pay, is $4 billion. What is the book net worth of the Ford Motor Company?

MR. WILLIS GOLDBECK: The aggregate liability of the Fortune 500 companies exceeds $2 trillion, which is roughly half a trillion more than the combined assets of the whole Fortune 500.

PROFESSOR ALAIN C. ENTHOVEN: I think it is important for people to understand this enormous issue here.

MR. JACK SHELTON: Ford Motor Company provides for our retirees and their eligible dependents health insurance and all kinds of related care for their lifetime. We also provide for surviving spouses and dependents of deceased employees who were eligible for retirement at the time of their death. At one time, when the economy was in a depressed state, for every person working we had one non-working person and his dependents insured so it was a one-to-one relationship. Now, with the economy back in a more normal state, it is something like 1.8 to 1.

MR. WILLIS GOLDBECK: This problem is most dramatic in steel and in oil. Bethlehem Steel now has one and a half covered retirees for every covered active worker. To give you a sense of the trend, ten and a half years ago Fortune 500 companies typically had twelve active workers for every covered retiree. Today, they have three or less.

4

Summary

I.

ALAIN C. ENTHOVEN, PH.D.

First of all, we certainly cannot predict the future. I agree with what Dr. Cooper and others have said, that attempts to do so can be useful exercises but they are not going to be literal prophecies. On the other hand, as Dr. Sammons and others have said, we can find some comfort in market forces if we let them work and if we have a little patience. So my diagnosis and prescription for this patient is basically that the patient is going to be okay. I recommend conservative treatment and a little patience. I am not at all persuaded that there will be a serious excess of doctors, and I do think there are serious quality problems that ought to be addressed.

We have heard a great deal of talk about supply and demand projections as if they were point estimates independent of market forces. We need to hear equally, or perhaps a little more than we have, about price and about the notion of economic equilibrium. In a normal market that is allowed to work, an excess supply can be only a temporary phenomenon. It drives down the price, which increases the amount demanded, and decreases the amount supplied until a new equilibrium is reached. In normal economic discourse, we think of the market as producing an equilibrium price at which the marginal valuations of consumers just equal the marginal costs of producers, and a kind of social optimum results.

It is very well known that such a normal market has not been allowed to operate in health care, at least for the past fifty years or so. The demand side for physicians' services has been robbed of cost consciousness by organized medicine's insistence on insurance arrangements based on the idea that every health care insurance scheme in a community must be open to participation by all physicians. The insured patient is not cost conscious because he is insured and does not have to pay. On the other hand, the insurer has no bargaining power because he has no legal right or authority to negotiate selectively or to direct patients to the contracting providers.

Until 1982 it was against the law in California for a health insurer to influence or participate in the patient's choice of provider in any way. That created a situation that Martin Feldstein characterized about fifteen years ago as "permanent excess demand"; physicians were able to create for themselves a gravity-free space independent of the forces of economic gravity. These principles of open-ended demand and free choice of provider have also prevented the development of private sector quality control.

Another important factor that has distorted the demand side has been open-ended subsidies by the government to the marginal cost of people's treatment decisions through Medicare/Medicaid and tax subsidies to private health insurance. When employers and employees anywhere in America decide that the employer will provide a hundred dollars more of health benefits, the federal government is, in effect, paying 40 percent of the cost. On the other hand, the supply side for physician services has also been strongly influenced by public policies and public subsidies. U.S. medical students, for instance, are not paying the full cost of their education. I am not necessarily saying that they should, just that the market is clearly not a free market.

I think that we are now moving rapidly, perhaps more rapidly than many of you realize, to a more cost-conscious demand side in which the payors are cost conscious because they are in price competition with other payors and in which they can negotiate for price with doctors. The demand side for doctors is being radically restructured. The most visible example of that is the rapid growth of health maintenance organizations, whose membership by last December, according to Dr. Ellwood's figures, reached 16.7 million, up 22 percent from the previous year. The previous year it had increased about 15 percent. Now, as Dr. Ellwood pointed out, a 15 percent per year compound growth rate would mean about sixty million HMO members by 1994 and 120 million by 1999. Professor Ginzberg assures us that that will not happen. He may be right about New York, but what Dr. Ellwood and I are talking about is America.

I think this growth in HMO membership will continue to accelerate or at least to maintain its 15 percent per year compound growth rate for several reasons. The first is the margin of economic advantage. Professor Newhouse found in a randomized controlled trial in Seattle, comparing Group Health Cooperative of Puget Sound with fee-for-service care there, that the Group Health Cooperative physicians did the job for about 28 percent less cost per person.

This process is going to be intensified by the fact that each time another million people leave the fee-for-service sector and go over to the HMOS, that leaves more doctors and more beds per capita to be supported in the fee-for-service sector, as well as significant adverse selection of providers. Mr. Shelton pointed out, I think very aptly, that it is likely to be the least efficient or the most costly providers who self-select to remain in the fee-for-service sector. There may also be a certain amount of adverse selection on the part of patients who are particularly attached to their fee-for-service providers.

Besides HMO growth, we now have preferred-provider insurance. I think that AB-3480 in California in 1982 was a signal event, comparable in health care finance to Proposition 13 in 1978 in public finances. The employers, labor, and the insurance industry lined up on one side and the California Medical Association on the other, and we came out with a new law which said that health insurers may negotiate and contract selectively with providers for alternative rates of payment and pass the savings on to their insureds. Preferred-provider insurance is now growing rapidly. As Mr. Shelton told us, employers are creating their own preferred-provider insurance plans. Hewlett-Packard is doing it and Ford Motor and General Motors are requiring their intermediaries to do it. It makes obvious sense for preferred-provider insurance schemes to be quality selective. I know that some of them are, at least at the level of identifying the doctors with bad records and making sure that they are not on the list.

The big four hospital corporations have bought their own insurance companies and are also marketing preferred-provider insurance. These organizations can and will develop the standards of physicians' performance that Dr. Wilbur recommends. This development has great potential and will radically change the whole demand side for physician services over the next decade.

Dr. Schwartz estimates that cost-contained demand would cut demand some 15 percent. That was a business-as-usual forecast which obviously does not allow for a radical restructuring of the health care system.

In Dr. Ellwood's scenario, in which HMOS and other efficient comprehensive care systems take care of their patients with one doctor for every 850 people, you can get a rather frightening prediction. That is, we are heading for a society with one doctor for every 400 people and the comprehensive care organizations will need one for every 800. Does that mean there will be a surplus? If so, what is the meaning of surplus? I think that we have been less precise about this than perhaps we ought to be. Does it mean, for example, physicians driving taxis? Frankly I doubt it. Does it mean that the market will not work, that prices for physician services just will not come down? I doubt that.

I think that competitive medical plans paying doctors $50,000 a year will drive competitive medical plans paying doctors $150,000 per year out of business. I think it is clear that we as a society have been paying more than we would need to in order to elicit the needed supply of well-qualified applicants to medical school. I think that the increased supply of doctors in this new cost-conscious competitive market is going to bring their incomes more into line with those of other professions with similar training and amount of work.

When I say into line, that needs to reflect such important factors as the postponement of the income-earning years. If you compare a factory worker earning $20,000 and a doctor earning $150,000, before you say the doctor earns seven times as much you need to bring it back to a present value at age eighteen and recognize that there is a lot of postponement of income for the doctor so that on the basis of the lifetime income stream those incomes are not nearly so different. You also need to reflect hours worked. There are probably a lot of doctors who, in terms of lifetime earnings, adjusted for postponement, are not earning a lot more than auto workers, and they probably will not suffer too much.

Another possible problem with a surplus would be that incomes might fall below the level needed to attract qualified applicants. In principle it would be easy for me to say this would be temporary and in the long run it would work out. Eventually the reduced supply would drive incomes back up, but that could be in a very long run. There are many potential compensatory mechanisms, however, if they are allowed to work. For one thing, physicians are gatekeepers. In these comprehensive care organizations, they can take back more and more of the work and redirect the dollars to themselves. For example, we may have physicians running intensive care units or even replacing nurse practitioners. When doctors earn $50,000 a year instead of $150,000 a year, there will be many tasks that they would be willing to do. We might even see prepaid group practice HMOS going to something like one doctor per 500 people instead of one per 800.

As Dr. Nicholson reminded us, there is the question of life-style. When your typical doctor has a husband who is also a doctor, forty hours of work each will support the family, even if each of these forty-hour work weeks is bringing in only $50,000. Then there is the question of the increasing number of women doctors; as Professor Reinhardt pointed out, their productivity is about 70 percent of that of male physicians. Yet another life-style compensatory factor might mean an earlier retirement.

Dr. Tarlov, talking about the use of time, mentioned leisure, more time with patients and so forth. I would add to his worthy list more time reading the literature and keeping up with this rapidly advancing science. Several speakers have commented on a major need for serious continuing medical education, where perhaps we would expect physicians to spend at least a half a day or a day a week in seminars, reading the literature, and in other similar activities. As Dr. Ottensmeyer very aptly pointed out, there is going to be a tremendous need for physicians in managerial tasks such as organizing and orchestrating services. Appropriately trained physicians would be the best qualified people to perform these tasks because they best understand what the services are all about.

Then there is expanding technology. The whole question of how many physicians we need is very technology-dependent. Mr. Whitehead mentioned a lot of doctor-saving technologies. I suggest that technology may also cut the other way. As Dr. Tosteson and Mr. Goldbeck and others pointed out, changing technology creates uncertainty and makes it even more difficult to predict the future.

Another compensatory factor is the serious strain on public finances which will inevitably lead to some cutback in public support for medical education. I do not think that this can be avoided. The shortfall in funds will have to be met by students and by the private sector and doubtless it will result in some downsizing in the medical education establishment. So, before joining the surplus bandwagon, I would want to hear full consideration of these compensatory mechanisms.

Now, this leaves Dr. Relman's very legitimate concern with the problem of Papa Doc U. I suggest that HMOS, preferred-provider insurance arrangements, and other competitive medical care plans will eventually solve that problem. It will take time, but such organizations have every incentive to pick very good U.S. medical graduates. The successful, sophisticated health care organizations understand that quality and economy go together. Having poor-quality doctors is not a good way to cut costs—poor-quality doctors lead to unsolved problems, complications, and increased costs. What will happen in the future is that Papa Doc U graduates will not be able to get jobs in the health care organizations. At the same time, more reasonable incomes will take some of the steam out of the pressure to become a doctor.

If we give it a little time, I think the invisible hand will take care of things just fine.

II
ARNOLD S. RELMAN, M.D.

The first issue we have tried to deal with is do we have, or are we going to have, a medical manpower problem and by that we have meant a total oversupply and/or a maldistribution. Some of us say no, some of us say yes, some of us are uncertain. I tend to agree with those who say that we will have, if we do not now have, a problem. I agree with my colleague, Dr. Petersdorf, that we now have too many of certain kinds of specialists relative to generalists and I agree with Dr. Tarlov's calculations, with or without the third compartment. The evidence is pretty clear that we are going to have more doctors than we need. We are, of course, a very large and heterogeneous country, and there are still big regional differences in manpower distribution, but that does not change the overall facts.

The next question is, Do we need to do something or will market forces solve the problem for us? Here I have the greatest sense of discomfort because I hear medicine being described as an industry and what we are involved in being described as a market, and many of us around this table have made the implicit assumption without any discussion that we can analyze this meaningfully in terms of the market. But I remind you that we began this discussion with a presentation by Dr. Anlyan in which he said, "Medical care is not a commodity or a luxury." We start with the assumption that it is an essential social service. If this is true, I do not see how we can rely mainly on market forces to determine the distribution of medical services or the numbers and kinds of doctors that we need. That is not to say that I am naive enough to believe that market forces have no effect or have had no effect in the past; they obviously do and they obviously will in the future, however imperfectly and slowly they may work.

The question, however, is not whether market forces can work, or have worked in the past, but rather as we plan ahead for the future should we allow them to work however they will, without regulation? And what would happen if we took that course? Now Professor Enthoven and, I gather, most economists say we should not worry; we should let the market work and then see where we are and things will probably work out. For the market to work in any sense, as I understand it, you need prudent buyers. Yet Dr. Tosteson said that a profession arises when buyers cannot be prudent. I think that is a profoundly true statement as it applies to the medical profession. The medical profession basically exists in economic terms because the buyers of health care cannot be prudent buyers but need the professional counsel and commitment of the medical profession to help them. So the special function of the medical profession is not just to provide expert services, but also to act as the trusted advisor and agent for the patient —not the customer or the client but the patient—who often cannot be a prudent buyer without the assistance of a physician. The quality and quantity of life itself often hinge on the assistance in a way that makes medical care different from any other necessity or commodity of life.

Professor Reinhardt and I have had a very long conversation in writing about whether medical care is in fact different from other commodities, particularly other essentials of life, and whether doctors are really basically different from businessmen. I have had similar discussions with leaders of the emerging for-profit, investor-owned, health care industry who insist that there is no basic difference between medical care and any other commodity and that doctors are basically businessmen. I am convinced that there are basic and irreducible and terribly important differences between what doctors do; what society expects them to do; what patients expect them to do; and what honest, conscientious, well-meaning businessmen are expected to do. Because of these differences, I do not think we can rely on market forces alone to solve the problem. If we allow the present situation to continue and we begin to get a large number of doctors, larger than we need to carry out their professional functions, we are going to do damage to the health care system. I believe we are already doing damage to the health care system. A cadre of underutilized physicians will really wreck the economy of the health care system and they will also do damage to the health of the American people. We will not only see the growth of expensive, unnecessary boutique medicine; we will also see lots of very bad medicine and we will see doctors doing things that they have no business doing.

Now Professor Enthoven and Dr. Ellwood and people who believe that organized institutions are going to provide health care and employ the doctors to do it say that the corporations will see to it that the quality of the physicians is okay, that the unqualified doctors will not be employed, and that health care will not only be efficient in terms of expense but also be relatively safe. Maybe that will happen, but as a physician I have the very uneasy feeling that, in order for us to serve the public needs in the best way, we need to maintain a certain amount of professional independence and autonomy. If we work for corporations, particularly for-profit corporations, we will not be able to work for our patients as well. The patients need to have us on their side as their purchasing agent, their counselor, their advisor, not as the employee of the corporation and certainly not as an investor in the corporation.

In the closed system in England that Dr. Lister told us about, where the physicians work for the state, many conditions of health care are regulated by the state, but what the state does not regulate is the professional practice of medicine. The doctors exercise their best professional judgment in the interest of their patients, using the resources they have available.

American medicine really faces a dilemma. We have to decide whether we accept the trend toward the corporate practice of medicine in which we become employees or co-venturers with the corporations in the practice of medicine, giving up our professional commitment to serve our patients first above everything else, or whether we will turn ultimately for salvation to the federal government. Dr. Tosteson says, and he is right, that the federal government has never subsidized anything that it did not regulate. If we accept a larger federal role in the provision of health care, we will have to accept increased regulation. This is a hard choice.

I keep thinking and hoping that there is a middle way, a way for the American medical profession to maintain its independence and its autonomy and still respond to the public's expectations of higher quality, better self-regulation, less expense, and more concern for the public interest than heretofore. It seems to me that we can begin with a few relatively uncomplicated initiatives. One is the initiative of U.S. foreign medical graduates. The political problem can be solved by taking it away from the states. The problem should be handled at the federal level with approved residency programs and a "grandfather" four-year phase-in time so that everybody already in the pipeline in foreign schools will be spared; that will remove much of the political heat. If we take the step we can reduce the number of mostly poorly trained physicians by about 2,500. I think that would be a great step forward.

The other things we can do also have to do with quality. We must eliminate residency programs that are not of high quality. We must look very closely at the pool of qualified students applying for medical school when we approve medical schools. Dr. Cooper and Dr. Sammons tell me that this is what the LCME does; I think it must be done more rigorously. We must do everything we can to reduce the number of marginal practitioners.

That will not be the whole solution, however, in my opinion. We must reduce the number of people coming out of medical school, and one of the ways to begin is by reducing the number of U.S. foreign medical graduates. I have no doubt, however, that we will ultimately have to reduce the number of graduates of U.S. medical schools as well. How we will do that is not clear to me from the discussions at this conference. I anticipate, however, that whether we like it or not, the federal government will probably have the last word.

III
J. ALEXANDER MCMAHON

In his opening comments, Dr. Anlyan noted that perceptions of the number of physicians needed over time has gone up and down, changing every ten or fifteen years, often because of external forces: Blue Cross, new perceptions, World War II, alternative delivery systems, cost containment, social justice, and so on. Most speakers echoed his caution about projections. Professor Newhouse did. Drs. Tarlov and Schwartz illustrated the problems by showing different projections, and Drs. Ellwood and Wilbur proved that you can take the same kinds of assumptions and get different results.

Dr. Anlyan closed by asking, first, Have we or will we have a surplus of physicians? and, second, If we have or will have, how do we correct the situation? With respect to the second question, Dr. Petersdorf offered a modest proposal with a heavy reliance on the benificent activities of the federal government, which raised the hair on my head and I am sure on some others. Dr. Schwarz told us the political difficulties of any reduction and Professor Havighurst showed us the problem with the law. Our conclusion about the second question is that there is not much we can do.

Do we have a surplus? I think the best answer came from Professor Reinhardt: beware of forecasts and before intervening let the market play out. There are many forces in motion that I suggest we cannot measure and I suspect if we try to measure them we will guess wrong. In contradistinction to Dr. Relman, I believe the market is better at self-correction. I think government-established policy is so often wrong that even when it is right it is likely to be changed in the near future.

Dr. Tarlov in his summary pointed out what I think is the right posture for now: forget the surplus issue and begin to dwell on what we do with respect to the numbers. What should we do in the medical schools? What does it mean for the practicing physicians and their organizations? What does it mean for better access to care and for Dr. Satcher's equity issue? What does it mean with respect to being able to deal with the inadequate training of USFMGS?

We are all familiar with the percentage of the GNP that goes to health care. We do not know, however, what percent goes to legal services or to transportation. Why? Because medical care comes out of two big pools, one government and one business, and they are the ones complaining about the increase in the percentage of GNP. I think that can change in time.

Index

Access, in North Carolina, 132
Accountability, demand for, 120
Accreditation requirements, alter to
    reduce manpower, 100
Admission requirements, tightening of,
    111
Affeldt, John E., 91
Alabama, licensing requirements, 68
Ambulatory sector, shift in care to, 20
Ambulatory surgery, 122
American Association of Retired
    Persons, 28
American Board of Internal Medicine,
    30
American College of Physicians,
    founded, 2
American College of Surgeons, 29;
    founded, 2
American Medical Association: found-
    ing of, 1; policy on studying
    medicine, 106; professional poll, 89
Anlyan, William G., 1–8, 11, 80, 128,
    134, 152, 155
Antitrust laws, 124
Applicants: quality of, 21; white male,
    50; women, 50
Area Health Education Centers (AHEC):
    developed, 6; purposes, 129
Arkansas, medical school applicants
    in, 50
Asper, Samuel P., 37–40, 82
Aspirations, of matching medical stu-
    dents, 61
Association of American Medical Col-
    leges: beginning of, 2; data on house

staff salaries, 103; efforts to alleviate
    doctor shortage, 9; policy on study-
    ing medicine, 106

Bethlehem Steel, working/retired ratio,
    145
Bevan, Arthur Dean, 3
Bigelow, Henry, 2
Blacks, education of, 50
Board of Medical Examiners, in North
    Carolina, 67
Boyle, Joseph F., 85, 87
Bureau of Health Manpower, 104
Bureau of Medical Quality Assurance,
    in California, 91
Business, concern with surplus of
    physicians, 136

Califano, Joseph, 13
California Medical Association, 149;
    manpower survey, 143
California: and FMGs, 90; medicine in,
    46
Canadians, in residency match, 60
Capitation decrease, effect on black
    applicants, 51
Cardiologists, 54
Care, quality of, 21
Career structure, in Great Britain, 73
Caribbean medical schools: effect on
    local economy, 40; FMGs from, 6; in
    residency match, 60
Carnegie Corporation, 2
Carnegie commission, 6; suggests
    increase in doctor supply, 5–6

Chiropractors, 49
Coggeshall report, 5
Colloton, John W., 83, 110
Colonial times, 1
Colorado, population/physician ratio in, 115
Columbia University, 1
Compartment: first, 15; second, 15; third, 17, 46; hours worked in, 47
Competition: among paramedicals, 110; among physicians, 82, 110
Congress, responds to doctor shortage, 9
Continuing medical education, 151
Cooper, John A. D., 50, 106, 147, 155
Coronary artery bypass surgery, rate of, 54
Corporate medical care, 134, 139; rise of, 113
Corporate providers, struggles among, 87
Cost management, 118
Council on Medical Education, 2
Credentialing responsibilities, of state licensing boards, 66
Credentials, fraudulent, 66

Danforth, William H., 55–59, 87, 94, 95
Debt: incurred in medical school, 41; business attitude toward, 123
Demand-based model, 14, 90
Dental schools, cutback in applicants, 57
Deregulation, Jacksonian era of, 1
Diagnosis Related Groups, 120
Disciplinary data bank, computerized, 69
Disciplinary responsibilities, of state licensing boards, 68
Distribution of physicians: geographic, 13, 23–27, 30, 95; of physicians in Great Britain, 95; specialty, 13, 30, 95; subspecialty, 30; uneven, 8
Drugs, sulfa: use of, 3
Duke Endowment, 3
Durenberger Bill, effect on residents' funding, 99
Durenberger, Senator, 84

Eavenson, C. Douglas, 136–137
Economic equilibrium, need for, 147
Educational Commission on FMGS, 15
Educational processes, need for study of, 59
Egdahl, Richard H., 48–49, 80, 144
Eliott, President, 2
Ellwood, Paul M., Jr., 15, 46–47, 53, 144, 148, 149, 155
Enthoven, Alain C., 53, 145, 147–52, 153

Family practitioners, surplus of, 49
Federal Trade Commission, 29
Federated Council of Internal Medicine, 31
Federation Licensing Examination (FLEX), 65
Fee structure, issue to be addressed, 82
Fee-for-service medicine: effect of HMOs on, 149; expected to grow, 144; practice, 15
Feldstein, Martin, 148
Fifth-pathway students, in residency match, 60
Fineberg, Harvey V., 80–82, 83, 88
First compartment, fee-for-service medicine, 15
Fitness, 121
Flexner report, challenged, 11, 56
Flexner, Abraham, 1910 study, 2
Ford Motor Company: creating own PPO insurance plan, 149; funding health care for retirees, 142; liability for retiree health care, 145
Forecasting: difficulties in medical manpower needs, 70; health manpower, 41
Foreign medical graduates (FMGS), 37–40, 135, 141; and ABIM, 100; in academe, 39; alien, in residency match, 61; backlash against, 82; in California, 91; and house staff reimbursement, 101; insurmountable problem, 111; market influences of, 37; in 1975, 6; numbers multiply, 4; participation in research, 39; as percentage of house staff, 98; political clout of, 7; problem in Great Britain, 71; in residency match, 61; training of, 33

Foreign medical schools, problem for state licensing boards, 66

Foundations, Rockefeller, 3

GMENAC commission: findings disputed, 19; findings of, 6, 90, 97; findings on target, 107; physician/population ratio, 46; revisited, 13–18; study, 80, 87, 107

Galusha, Bryant L., 64–69, 86, 95, 135, 141–42

General Medical Council, 71

General Motors, creating own PPO insurance plan, 149

General practitioners, 26; in Great Britain, 73

Genetic engineering, 119

Geographic distribution, 13; of physicians, 23–27

Ginzberg, Eli, 48, 87, 91, 107, 140–41, 144, 148

Goldbeck, Willis, 51–52, 118–24, 138, 145, 151

Goodenough Committee, in Great Britain, 77

Government, federal: and funding medical system, 87

Government, state: role in medical education, 127

Graduate Medical Education, Accreditation Council on, 31

Graduate medical education requirement: as an exercise in discrimination, 65; assures quality, 64

Graettinger, John S., 60–63, 64, 65, 81, 82, 94

Grandfathering, antitrust implications, 126

Great Britain: closed system in, 154; medical costs in, 89; medicine in, 70–79

Great Society, 5, 6

Grenada, St. George's medical school in, 98

Group practice, multispecialty, 49

Guadalajara, FMGS from, 6

Hanlon, C. Rollins, 28–30, 135

Harvard Medical School, 1; workshop on medicine/personal relations, 35

Havighurst, Clark C., 124–27, 138, 140, 141, 156

Health care professionals, nonphysician, 144

Health insurance, 148

Health maintenance organizations (HMOS), 18; and skimming healthy population, 53; changing physician attitude toward, 119; enrollment in Los Angeles, 46; growth of, 144; rapid growth of, 148

Health Manpower Act, 6

Health Policy Agenda for the American People, 142

Health Professions Educational Act, legislation passed, 5

Heckler, Margaret, 137

Hewlett-Packard, creating own PPO insurance plan, 149

Hill-Burton Act, 4

Hospital corporations, and insurance, 149

Hospital trustees, effect on medical care quality, 48

Hospitals: for polio, 4; for tuberculosis, 4; incentives to reduce training programs, 100

House staff: excess causes physician surplus, 105; funding of training, 105; programs, 99; size of, 102; stipends of, 101

Hungary, invasion of, 5

Immigration and Naturalization Service, 38

Income: and physician surplus, 44; for physicians, 81; of physicians, 134

Individual Retirement Accounts (IRAS), 14

Industry: relations with insurance companies, 123; role in determining physician numbers, 118; to provide support for medical research, 121

Institute of Medicine, 6

Insulin, discovery of, 3

Insurance companies: for non-HMO physicians in California, 47; relations with industry, 123

Internal medicine, inadequate numbers of physicians in, 31

International health service corps, suggestion for, 138
International medicine, drawbacks for young physicians, 143
Iowa, 84

Jacksonian era, 1
Japan, health care in, 143
Johns Hopkins, founding of, 2
Journals, scientific, 120

Kaiser (HMO), 46
Keogh plans, 14
Kerr, Clark, on Carnegie Commission, 91
Kidney stone removal, in Great Britain, 89
King, Martin Luther, 114
Kings College, 1
Koch, 2

Lansteiner, performs first blood transfusion, 2
Laparotomy, first, 1
Law school, in St. Louis, 56
Law, 124
Legal system, and medical licensing boards, 142
Legislative perspective, 9–10
Legislature, state: choices regarding public medical schools, 132; and physicians' licensing in Massachusetts, 80; role in reducing physician numbers, 48
Leisure time, use of by physicians, 92
Licensing boards, state, 64
Licensure: by endorsement/reciprocity, 67; state control over, 80; of concern to industry, 122
Life expectancy, of black men, 137
Life-style: effect on physician income, 151; of physicians, 34; of young physicians, 144; physician, 7
Limited licensed practitioners, 110
Lister, Joseph, 1
Lister, John S., 70–79, 87, 91, 95, 154
Lithotripter, effect on costs, 89
Little Rock, riots, 5
Long, Crawford, 1

Longevity, effect on medical profession, 123

McDowell, Ephraim, 1
McMahon, J. Alexander, 155–56
Magnuson, Senator, 117
Mahoney, Margaret, 49–50, 90, 91
Maldistribution: by specialty, 105, 117; geographic, 117
Malpractice, 121
Management efficiency, emphasized in Great Britain, 70
Managerial positions, for physicians, 151
Market forces, effect on physician excess, 152
Marriages, dual-career, 35
Massachusetts General Hospital, 1
Massachusetts, prenatal care under Medicaid, 80
Maternity leave, for physicians, 35
Mayer, Eugene S., 92, 127–33, 139
Medicaid, 5
Medical Practice Act, 141
Medical care: accessibility to, 107; as a commodity, 153; defined, 152; federal role equals more regulation, 154; restructuring of, 141
Medical economics, need for more exposure to, 57
Medical education fund, 103
Medical education: how to determine quality of, 120; public, 115; quality of, 86; role of state government in, 127; shortcomings in, 57; university's role in, 55
Medical history, need for more exposure to, 57
Medical industry, 93
Medical management, 135
Medical profession, differs from medical industry, 93
Medical school: alternatives to, 50; boards of trustees, 115; class size and house staff size, 100; class size in, 13, 93, 115, 116; as public service corporation, 11
Medical school applicants: must be scrutinized, 155; numbers decreasing, 112

Medical school class size: cut back to control physician excess, 124; no need to reduce, 112
Medicare, 5
Medicine: alternatives to, 50; bizarre forms of, 94
Medicine, corporate, 119
Meharry Medical School, 51
Mental health, area needing more physicians, 119
Millis commission, supports family practice specialty, 5
Minorities, education of, 50
Model: demand-based, 14; need-based, 14
Money: effect on practice patterns; at root of physician surplus question, 141
Morbidity patterns, from epidemiological models, 41
Moser, Robert H., 30–33, 52
Moynihan, Daniel Patrick, 51
Multitier care, 122
Myocardial infarctions, rate of, 53

National Board of Medical Examiners, licensing examination by, 65
National Health Service, in Great Britain, 70, 95
National Health Service Corps, 33, 52, 138; founded, 6; intent of legislation, 52; scholarship discontinuation and blacks, 51
National Institutes of Health, 4; FMGS on staff of, 39
National Medical Association, 137
Need-based model, 14, 90
Nesbitt, Tom E., 53, 89
New York City, medical expenditures in, 48
Newhouse, Joseph P., 23–27, 82, 128, 149, 155
Nicholson, Britain, 34–36, 89, 123, 144, 151
Nixon administration, requests increase in doctors, 5
Nonphysician providers, 49; growth in, 53; in GMENAC study, 53
Nonwhite health, poorer than health of whites, 137

North Carolina: physicians and legislators, 92; spontaneous oral exam for licensing, 68
Nurse midwife, in GMENAC study, 53
Nurse practitioner, 49; in GMENAC study, 53

Ohio, attempts to close medical school, 108
Ophthalmology, specialty society founded, 2
Optometrists, 49; in GMENAC study, 53
Oregon: medical school applicants in, 50; oral examination requirement for license, 67
Osteopathic schools, class size in, 13
Osteopaths: enrollment assumptions in GMENAC, 14; in residency match, 60
Ottensmeyer, David J., 134–35, 151

PGY-1 positions, excess of, 60
Papa Doc University, 83, 151
Pasteur, Louis, 2
Penicillin, discovery of, 3
Pennsylvania, University of, 1
Petersdorf, Robert G., 49, 90, 97–105, 109, 130, 140, 143–44, 152, 155
Physician extender, 129
Physician income: in relation to union employees, 90; may equal other professionals', 150; reaching plateau, 134
Physician shortage, 9, 94
Physician surplus, 20–22, 119, 124, 152; AMA position on, 109
Physician/population ratio: in Great Britain, 70; history of, 6; in Los Angeles today, 46; metropolitan, 24; nonmetropolitan, 24; in North Carolina, 128
Physicians' roles, changes in, 113
Physicians: College of, founded, 2; deviant, 68; employment practices of, 12; function in the economy, 113; as social instrument, 11; specialty choices of, 12; work hours, 47
Physicians, women: productivity of, 13
Plastic surgery, 48
Podiatrists, 49

Poor, health care of, 8
Population growth, nonoccidental in United States today, 52
Population/physician ratio, 115; in North Carolina, 131; sectional differences in, 42
Postponement, of income-earning years by physicians, 150
Practitioner, solo, 47
Preferred-provider insurance, 149
Preventive medicine, 121
Primary care physician, ratio to specialist, 102
Priorities in medical care, emphasized in Great Britain, 70
Professional schools, for older Americans, 52
Projections of physician supply, in GMENAC, 18
Providers, limited-license: supported by business, 123

Quality, assessing in physicians, 136
Quality care, 21; licensing boards' effect on, 64
Quotas, AMA opposition to, 109

Regionalization of services, preferred by business community, 120
Reinhardt, Uwe E., 41–45, 81, 151, 153, 156
Relman, Arnold S., 83, 86, 87, 88, 140, 151, 152–55, 156
Research, medical: by industrial companies, 85
Residencies, first-choice, 81; unmatched, 88
Residency Review committees, 29; set tougher standards, 31; requirements for residency programs, 100
Residency matching program, 60; nonmatches in, 82
Residency programs, eliminate those of low quality, 155
Residency requirement, for LCME graduates, 144
Residency training programs, 60–63; need reappraisal, 139; in internal medicine, 16
Resource Allocation Working Party, 95

Retirees, health care costs for industry, 142
Retirement age, estimate in GMENAC report, 14
Retirement, considered by GMENAC, 13
Rockefeller Foundation, 3
Rogers, Paul G., 9–10, 28, 52, 87, 88
Royal College of Physicians, 70

Sammons, James H., 88, 109–12, 114, 119, 135, 142, 143, 155
Satcher, David, 50–51, 52, 136, 137–38, 140, 143, 156
Schwartz, William B., 19–22, 149, 155
Schwarz, M. Roy, 115–18, 156
Second compartment, federal medical employees, 15
Self-care, 121, 145; effect on medical care, 84
Selman v. Harvard Medical School, 125
Senior Registrar Training Committee, in Great Britain, 76
Shelton, Jack K., 49, 142–43, 145
Sherman Act, 140; favors competition, 124
Shift work, trend toward, 34
Short Report, in Great Britain, 77
Shortage of doctors, 9
Size of town, critical, 24
Sloan, Frank, 19
Space medicine, 119
Specialists, ratio to primary care physicians, 102
Specialties, competition among, 25
Specialty: distribution, 13; maldistribution in, 49; training, 126
Specialty boards, and manpower supply, 100
Sputnik, 5
Staff privileges, withholding, 127
State licensing boards, strengthening of, 111
Status of physicians, 138
Stevens, Rosemary A., 11–12, 82, 86, 139–40
Stipends, residents', 17
Student loans, seen as an opportunity, 138
Study of Internal Medicine Manpower, 97

Subspecialization rate, 17
Subspecialties, undersubscribed: funding for, 32
Sulfa drugs, use of, 3
Surgeons: American College of, 2, 29; non-board-certified, 97; surplus of in some communities, 48
Surgery, ambulatory, 122
Surplus, physician, 20–22; economic definition of, 44; effects of, 21; is there one? 8; may not exist in internal medicine, 31

Tarlov, Alvin R., 13–18, 46, 48, 53, 63, 81, 92, 151, 152, 155, 156
Technology: effect on future physicians, 151; as a potent factor needing consideration, 84
Telecommunications: impact on physicians' practices, 30; part of medical information explosion, 120
Texas: licensing requirements, 67; medical school applicants in, 50
Third compartment, prepaid care, 17
Third-party payment, 118
Todd Commission, in Great Britain, 77
Tosteson, Daniel C., 77, 93, 94, 112–14, 134, 138, 139, 144–45, 151, 153, 154
Toxicology, specialty needing more physicians, 119
Training programs: funding in industrial setting, 94; in Great Britain, 76
Transplantation, beginning of, 5
Truman Commission, 4
Tuition increase: effect on black applicants, 51; as method of controlling manpower planning, 41

Unemployment, medical: in Great Britain, 77
United States, work by physicians outside, 123

USFMGS: policy requires articulation, 139; a political problem, 83; rejected at U.S. medical schools, 88; in residency match, 61; rights of, 86; Mr. Rogers's solution, 87; solve at federal level, 156
University of California, efforts to reduce house staff in, 99
University of Pennsylvania, 1

Veterans Administration, effect of changes in, 10
Veterans, medical care of, 10
Visa Qualifying Examination, effect on FMGS, 61

Washington University, graduate education at, 56
Washington, population/physician ratio in, 116
Waste, much to be cut, 119
Weinberger, Caspar, as Secretary of HEW, 6
Weiskotten commission, 3
Wellness, as a new field, 48
Wellness programs, within business community, 119
Whitehead, Edwin C., 84, 145, 151
Wilbur, Richard S., 47, 135–36, 139, 149, 155
Willink Committee, in Great Britain, 77
Women physicians: effect on practice patterns, 34; in Great Britain, 71; in part-time practice, 35; productivity of, 13, 44, 151
Women: medical students at Meharry, 51; in medicine, 7
World War II, effect on doctor supply, 3
Writing skills, weak in physicians, 57
Wroblewski, Rita, 138–39

Yale Medical School, 1

Library of Congress Cataloging-in-Publication Data
Private Sector Conference (10th : 1985 : Duke University
Medical Center)
How many doctors do we need?
(Duke Press Policy Studies)
Includes index.
1. Physicians—United States—Supply and demand—
Congresses. 2. Physicians, Foreign—United States—
Supply and demand—Congresses. 3. Medical education—
United States—Congresses. 4. Medical policy—United
States—Congresses. 1. Yaggy, Duncan. 11. Hodgson,
Patricia, 1942—   . [DNLM: 1. Education, Medical—
United States—congresses. 2. Forecasting—congresses.
3. Health Policy—United States—congresses.
4. Physicians—supply and distribution—United States—congresses.
W3 PR945F 10th 1985h / W 76 P961 1985h]
RA410.7.P75 1985 331.12'9161'069520973 85-31097
ISBN 0-8223-0577-1